THE PRACTICAL GUIDE TO

magnet therapy

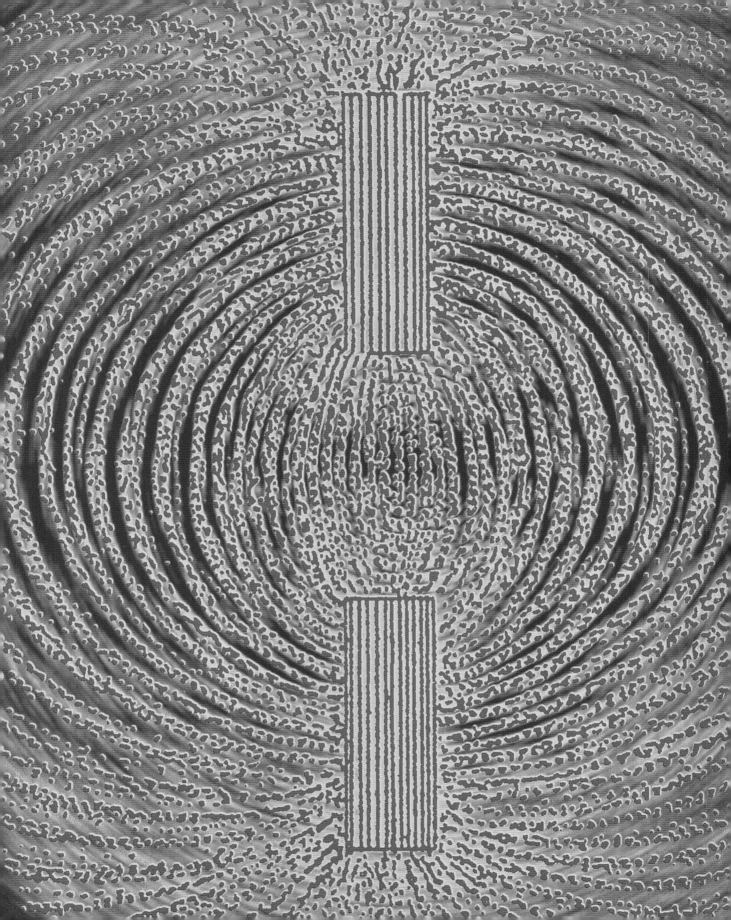

THE PRACTICAL GUIDE TO

magnet therapy

Peter Rose FSI

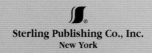

Sterling Publishing Co., Inc.
New York

Library of Congress Cataloging-in-Publication Data Available

10 9 8 7 6 5 4 3 2 1

Published in 2001 by Sterling Publishing Company, Inc.

387 Park Avenue South, New York, NY 10016

© 2001 Godsfield Press

Text © 2001 Peter Rose

Peter Rose asserts the moral right to be identified as the author of this work.

Distributed in Canada by Sterling Publishing

c/o Canadian Manda Group, One Atlantic Avenue, Suite 105

Toronto, Ontario, Canada M6K 3E7

Distributed in Australia by Capricorn Link (Australia) Pty Ltd

PO Box 6651, Baulkham Hills, Business Centre, NSW 2153, Australia

Note from the publisher

Any information given in this book is not intended to be taken as a replacement for medical advice.

Any person with a condition requiring medical attention should consult a qualified doctor or therapist.

Every effort has been made to ensure that all the information in this book is accurate.

However, due to differing conditions, tools, and individual skills, the publisher cannot be responsible for any injuries,

losses, and other damages which may result from the use of the information in this book.

Printed and bound in China

ISBN 0-8069-2777-1

The publishers wish to thank the following for the use of pictures:
The Art Archive: p. 97; A–Z Botanical Collection: p. 72; Corbis: p. 20;
Fortean Picture Library: p. 81; Garden Picture Library: p. 87;
Getty One Stone: pp. 36, 38, 41, 44, 50, 64, 65, 80, 102;
Image Bank: pp. 17, 19, 21, 42, 54, 62, 79, 84:
NASA: pp. 30, 76; Science Photo Library: pp. 2, 10, 14, 22, 56, 90.
Front cover photograph by Bill Milne

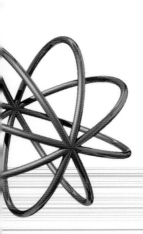

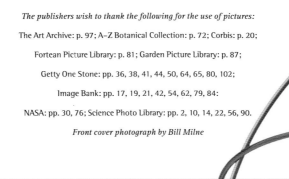

✳ | Contents

Introduction   6

How to use this book   8

Chapter one / History and background   10

Chapter two / Using magnets   32

Chapter three / Specific healing   54

Chapter four / Magnetic influences   76

Chapter five / Applying the theory   94

Glossary   122

Useful suppliers   124

Index   126

Acknowledgments   128

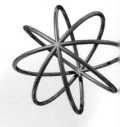

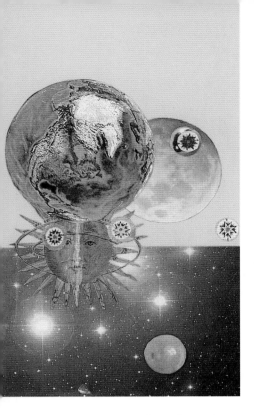

The forces of magnetism affect the world we live on, and reach out far into the solar system. The earth itself has its own magnetic field, while the field around the moon influences the pull of the tides.

Every living thing gives out an electrical field or an aura. Imbalances in this can be healed using a variety of alternative therapies, including crystal healing.

Introduction

The aim of this book is to explore the phenomenon of magnetism and its effects on the energy flows within our bodies and our living environments, and to examine how it can be used to improve our emotional and physical health.

Magnetism itself is discussed in detail—what it is, how it works—and its history as a tool for navigation and for healing is covered in depth. Magnetism is all around us; it is part of our natural world and has a significant effect on us and our environment. With the invention of electromagnetism, a new source of magnetic force has become available. Electromagnetism is the basis of modern technology, and in today's world we are constantly being bombarded with electromagnetic forces, sometimes with undesirable consequences. But electromagnetism has also brought great advances in the fields of modern medicine and magnet therapy. We now have devices that can control and manipulate the flows of magnetic forces and adjust them to treat specific ailments or injuries. We will discuss this new technology and see how it is used in magnet therapy.

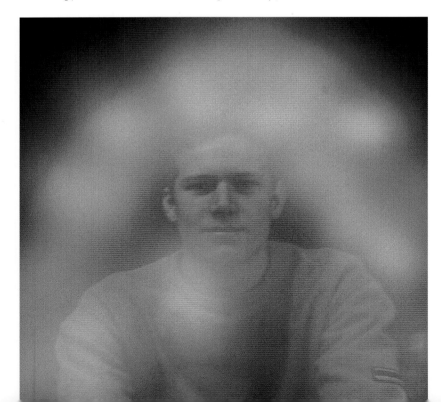

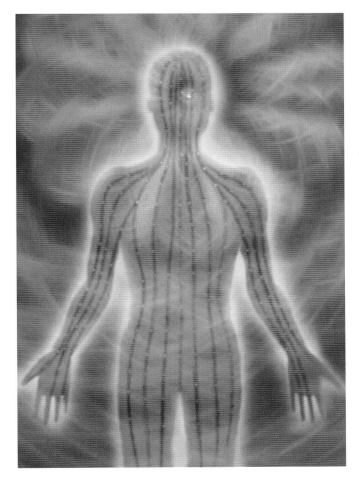

The internal life force—chi or qi—flows around the body on pathways called meridians. This flow of energy can be improved by the application of magnets to particular points on the body.

A Lo Pau pa kua compass, used in the ancient Chinese art of feng shui. This practice works with the earth's natural vibrations to ensure a positive flow of energy.

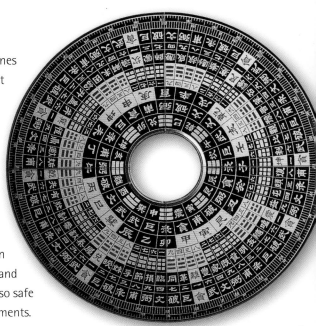

Magnet therapy can be used to control pain, stop infection, heal bones and scar tissue, rejuvenate cells, and balance the body's energy levels. It can also be effectively combined with most other therapies. The application of suitable strength magnets to the body can have many beneficial physiological effects. Magnets can increase blood and oxygen circulation, along with the nutrient-carrying potential of the blood; they are able to speed up the healing of nervous tissue and bones; they can powerfully influence the production of certain hormones; and they can stimulate and foster enzyme activity and other related physiological processes.

Small magnets on adhesive pads can be purchased for use on specific, smaller areas of the body, while flexible magnetic strips and supports can be bought for use on larger areas. Magnet therapy is also safe enough to be used on animals and pets, and can treat a number of ailments.

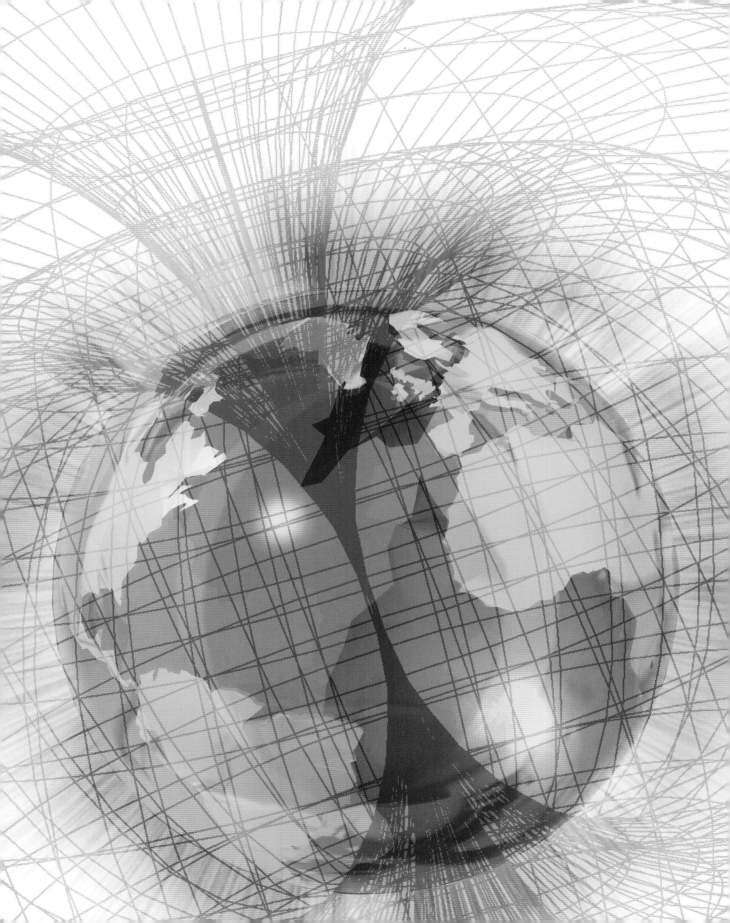

How to use this book

This comprehensive and lavishly illustrated book discusses magnets, electro-magnetism, and how magnet therapy can be used for healing purposes. This unique book has adopted a truly holistic approach, so there are also examples of how magnets can be used with other forms of therapy to relieve the symptoms of illness and improve recovery times. Simple and readable, without pretension or complication, but still giving a full explanation of the forces involved in magnetism, this book is both an introduction to this subject for those new to alternative medicine and a valuable tool for those who are already involved in any form of natural therapy.

Chapter one: this chapter introduces you to magnetism and its history. It also describes electromagnetism and looks at its role in modern medicine and alternative therapies.

Chapter two: this is a detailed discussion of the human body and the way in which our body systems and organs work, and how they are affected by magnets and the practice of magnet therapy.

Chapter three: more detail is gone into in this chapter as specific ailments and the effect that magnets have on them are discussed. There are also instructions for self-help exercises in this section.

Chapter four: this chapter looks at other aspects of magnetism, such as its role in folklore and its influence in our dreamworld, and also at how magnet therapy works in conjunction with other alternative therapies, such as homeopathy, flower essences, shiatsu, and acupuncture.

Chapter five: in this section a brief overview is given of the five transformations, and how they are relevant to magnet therapy. Meridians and acupuncture points are also discussed, and there are numerous charts to help you locate the correct acupuncture point for your particular ailment.

This book is an exploration of the positive power of magnetism. It deals with the history of magnets, their myths and folklore, and their ability to speed up the healing process. This is an instructive and useful book for amateur and professional alike, whatever your interest in magnets.

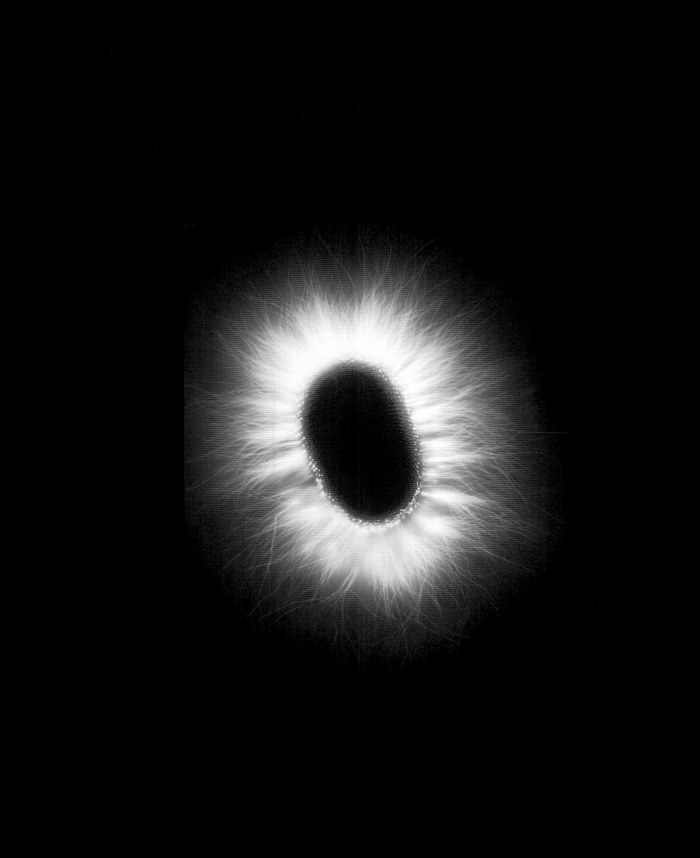

Chapter one

History and background At one time, magnetism was thought to be a kind of magic and ancient civilizations regarded this power to attract objects with wonderment. Gradually, new information replaced this wonder and amazement with hard facts and scientific explanation. With this new knowledge came a familiarity with these hitherto mysterious forces, and the healing power of magnetic forces came to be disregarded. Some specialists have kept this tradition alive, however, and with the exploration of new advances in the field of magnets, electromagnetic devices are being developed to take the use of variable magnetic fields to new heights. There is still much to be gained from the study of magnets and their powers, and with old science working side by side with new technology, great advances can be predicted in the world of complementary and orthodox medicine and healthcare.

✳ | What is magnetism?

GRAVITY AND MAGNETISM

Gravity, like magnetism, involves an unseen energy force that influences objects within that field of energy. The tides of the ocean are influenced by the gravitational pull of the moon. So what is the actual difference between gravity and magnetism?

The dictionary says magnetism is the property of attraction displayed by magnets, while gravity is said to be the force that attracts matter to the center of the earth. A gravitational field is the area of force surrounding a body of finite mass, in which another body would experience an attractive force that is proportional to the product of the masses and inversely proportional to the distance between them. A magnetic field is defined as an area of force surrounding a permanent magnet or a moving charged particle that acts directly on iron objects or on other magnets placed in the force field. The planet earth has a sufficiently large mass to have a gravitational field and has sufficient magnetic material within its body to have a magnetic field.

Magnetism refers to the ability of certain objects to exert an unseen force on another object. This pulling power of the magnet is unusual in that it is not reduced (within normal timescales and operational conditions) when its energy is released. One of the basic laws of physics is that energy can be neither created nor destroyed, only transformed. This usually means that energy gets transferred from one state to another or from one object to another; but a magnet keeps its ability to be a magnet even after it has influenced another object.

MOLECULAR MAGNETS

Each molecule of matter can be seen as a tiny magnet. Molecules of some materials, such as iron, have greater magnetic abilities than others, such as wood. Magnetism in metals is caused by the alignment of all the molecules and atoms in such a way as to make them work together and pull in the same direction; they unite to influence other objects. When a piece of iron is not magnetized, its molecules are all pulling in random directions, each one counteracting its neighboring molecules. Magnetic forces cause the molecules of a substance to line up in the same way relative to each other. In some cases, this causes the whole substance whose molecules are being aligned to become magnetic. When the molecules are all lined up in the same direction, they can begin to exert a considerable influence on other objects around them.

MAGNETIC POLES

The two ends of a magnet, where the force is concentrated, are known as the poles of the magnet. When a magnet is used as a compass, one end swings north; this is called the north, or north-seeking, pole. If you cut a bar magnet in two you end up with two complete magnets, each with a north and a south pole.

A fundamental law of magnetism is that opposite poles attract and like poles repel. If you remember this, everything will make sense. The magnetic force exerted between the poles of two different magnets is said to follow the "inverse square law," which means that if you double the distance between the poles of two different magnets the force is reduced to a quarter of its previous strength. So the force is greatly reduced the farther away from the magnet you go.

ELECTROMAGNETISM

Electromagnetism refers to the magnetic forces that are produced by electricity. Electromagnetic devices can be manipulated and controlled to produce magnetic influences that vary in strength and direction. This is a relatively new application of magnetic energy, but it is now all-pervasive and can have the same effect on us as natural magnetic forces. We shall be looking at electromagnetism and its use in magnet therapy later in the book (see pages 20–21).

DIFFERENT MAGNETIC MATERIALS

Different materials have different abilities that enable them to become magnets. There are four classes of modern commercial magnets, each based on its material composition. Within each class is a family of grades, which classify the strength of the magnet, i.e. strong, medium, weak, with their own magnetic properties. These four classes are neodymium iron boron, samarium cobalt, ferrite, and alnico. Neodymium iron boron and samarium cobalt are collectively known as rare-earth magnets because they are both composed of materials from the rare earth group of elements. Neodymium iron boron ($Nd_2Fe_{14}B$) is the most recent commercial addition to the collection of modern magnetic materials. At room temperature, neodymium iron boron magnets exhibit the strongest magnetic pull of all materials. Samarium cobalt is made in two compositions, SM_1Co_5 and Sm_2Co_{17}, and these are often referred to as SmCo 1-5 or SmCo 2-17 types.

Ferrite magnets, also known as ceramic magnets, were developed in the 1950s and are still in general use today. (Ferrite magnets are made by subjecting a ferrite material to an electromagnetic field of a sufficient strength and for a sufficient duration to leave a residual magnetic effect.) A special form of ferrite magnet is the "flexible" material, made by bonding ferrite powder into a flexible binder, such as rubber or fabric. Alnico magnets (chemical formula AlNiCo) were made commercially in the 1930s and are still used extensively today.

Magnetic rubber is produced by heavily loading ferrite powder of a barium or strontium base into a rubber or PVC matrix and extruding it into the required shape or calendering it into thin strips. The material is then usually magnetized in a secondary operation. Most forms of rubberized magnets are flexible.

MAGNETIC MEASUREMENTS

Magnetism is like a collection of lines of force: the strength of that force is known as flux density. This is the concentration of lines of force per unit area passing from one pole to the other. Flux density is measured in teslas per square meter or in the older gauss units. (Although tesla units are more up to date, all of the magnets throughout this book are measured in gauss. This is because the magnets and magnetic equipment most readily available for the purposes described here are measured in gauss, and will therefore be more recognizable.)

Magnets come in all kinds of shapes, sizes, and colors. The magnets pictured are all designed to be used safely on the body.

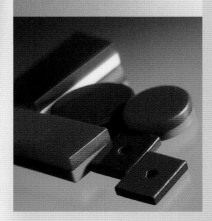

✳ | How magnets affect the human body

MAGNETIC POLES

In magnet therapy the poles are referred to as negative or positive. Some simplify things further by referring only to a color for each side of a magnet, usually red or blue. It is helpful to memorize the pole attributes. A north-seeking pole is positive and red. This may be marked as "N" on old magnets. It is sometimes called the "yang" side. A south-seeking pole is negative and blue (some texts may refer to it as the green side). This may be marked as "S" on old magnets. It is sometimes called the "yin" side. Generally in magnet therapy, a positive (red) side will stimulate, and a negative (blue) side will sedate or calm.

Magnets create order among chaotically intermingled molecules, and thereby improve the ability of these molecules to flow through narrow tubes; this has important implications for the human body.

We can compare the flow of molecules within a blood vessel with the flow of logs down a river. If all the logs are lined up in the same direction, they will flow smoothly along with the river and reach their destination. If they get out of line with each other, they become entangled and jam the flow of the other logs. Magnets ensure that the molecules are lined up in the same direction, all facing down the river. Similar comparisons can be made when considering the flows of energy, or life forces, around the body: chaos slows things down; order speeds things up.

Research has indicated that magnets support the formation of amino acids and have a positive influence on the metabolism of the body. In other words, magnets can increase the speed at which your body does the good things it needs to do, i.e. bring blood and oxygen to an injury site, in order to repair any damage it has suffered. However, magnets can also have a negative effect in this context: it is important never to use magnets on open wounds or freshly torn muscles as the increased flow of blood in these cases is dangerous.

Water makes up an astonishing 66 percent of our bodies. Magnets weaken the surface strength of water, making it easier for anything carried by the water to cross over to cells where it may be needed. Hemoglobin, the oxygen-carrying

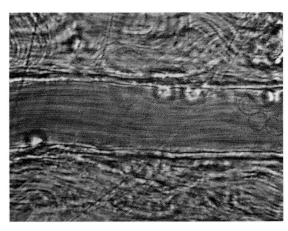

The blood flow through a vessel can be accelerated and improved with the careful use of magnets. This can mean that an injury will heal much more efficiently.

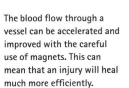

substance in red blood-cells, contains iron, which fixes oxygen and takes it where it is needed. If these iron particles are lined up, they create an accumulation of energy that strengthens the blood.

Furthermore, magnets can influence molecules of the body without actually touching them. This means that a magnet placed on the body can affect the cells and fluids below the skin surface, without the need to puncture the skin.

THE MOBILIZING EFFECTS OF MAGNETS

Magnets have an organizing, enhancing, and encouraging ability rather than a direct or combative action. They work by improving the flow of energy and fluids. Magnets themselves do not directly fight viruses or the invasion of toxins, but they do encourage the body's own natural defense energies to be more active. Some initial research has suggested that very powerful magnetic fields can affect cancerous growths, but further investigation is required.

A WORD OF WARNING
Very strong electromagnetic forces can cause severe damage to the human body. People who work with electromagnetic equipment such as large radio transmitters take careful precautions. The potentially adverse effects of magnetic and electromagnetic "pollution" from such things as power transmission lines is the cause of some concern.

Magnet therapy can be used in conjunction with physical therapies, such as shiatsu, as well as with other therapies.

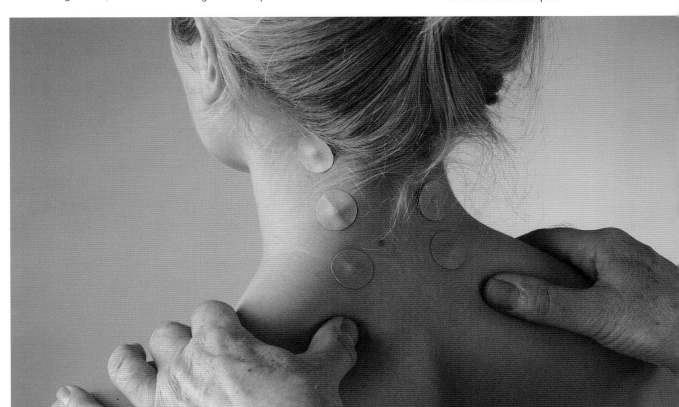

The history of magnet therapy

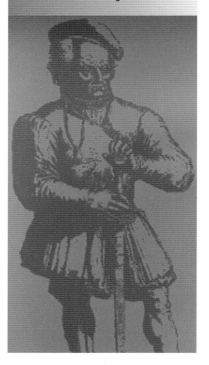

Magnetism has been around since the Big Bang and the creation of matter, so it is as old as the universe itself. There is no evidence that magnets were used by the earliest humanoid life forms. However, there have been claims that the most primitive ancestors of humans had built-in magnets in their nasal cavity, which enabled them to find their way around—archeological evidence has shown that the nasal cavities of some fossils have exhibited faint magnetic traces.

We do know that the magnetic properties of certain materials were known to the ancient Chinese. In the book entitled *Herbal of Divine Farmer*, which dates from the Han dynasty (about 200 BCE), there is a reference to magnets being used to relieve swollen joints. The ancient Chinese almost certainly used magnets and magnetic material to try to improve the flow of chi or qi (internal energy or life force that flows around channels or meridians in the body). The Chinese have also been credited with inventing the compass in the middle of the first century, while others claim it didn't come into use until the second century AD.

The Roman historian Pliny the Elder (23–79) recorded the treatment of eye diseases with magnets. The Persian physician Avicenna (980–1037) used magnets to relieve depression. The ancient Sanskrit text, the *Atharvaveda*, refers to the use of magnets to stop bleeding. Egyptian records indicate that magnets were part of their healing methods; it is said that Cleopatra used to wear a small magnet on her forehead with the intention of preserving her looks. The Vikings from Nordic Europe are said to have used a magnetic rock, known as a lodestone, on their sea voyages as a navigational aid—a forerunner of the compass today.

It is said that Elizabeth I of England (1533–1603) used magnets to improve her health on the advice of her famed physician Dr. William Gilbert. Some claim that it was William Gilbert who discovered that the properties of a lodestone could be transfered to an ordinary piece of iron by rubbing it with the lodestone. He was allegedly the first person to suggest that a compass always points to the north. The Austrian physician and founder of mesmerism, Franz Mesmer (1734–1815), experimented with therapeutic treatments that used magnets. The German physician Samuel Hahnemann (1755–1843), the founder of homeopathic medical practices, was a great advocate of the use of magnets in the healing process, and often used them in combination with his homeopathic remedies.

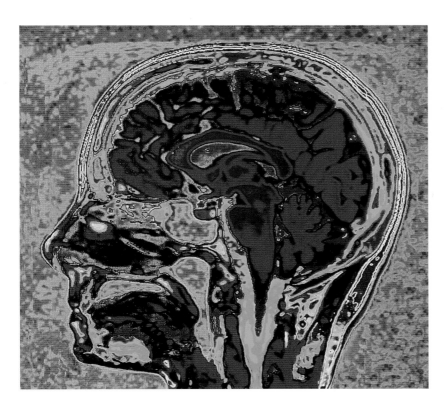

MRI machines are able to provide a detailed cross-section of any body part. They show soft tissue structures, as well as bone.

The magnetic properties of a lodestone can be transferred to a piece of metal just by rubbing it.

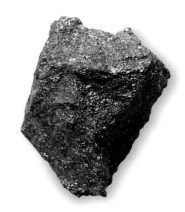

Today, every high-tech hospital routinely uses electromagnetic equipment. Magnetic Resonance Imaging (MRI) machines analyze the rates of absorption of high-frequency radio waves by the water molecules in tissues that have been placed in a strong magnetic field. MRI machines build up a set of computerized cross-sectional drawings that are similar to X-rays but do not have the same frequency of wave form and do not only show "hard" objects (such as bone). An MRI scan can be used to look at soft tissue structures and locate tumors. The absorption rate is the constantly varying ability of tissue to absorb magnetic forces and not reflect back the waves or pulses of energy. Microwave therapy uses extremely short wave-length electromagnetic impulses. These are very high frequency, high intensity, and strongly focused. We may have come a long way from lodestones to MRI, but magnetism is the foundation of all these advances.

✳ | Invisible energy

VIBRATING CRYSTALS

Crystals have a specific internal structure and an external shape in which plane faces intersect at definite angles. They have the power to oscillate or vibrate at constant frequencies. These vibrations may be too subtle for us to detect with our physical senses but it is true that they do exert an influence over us.

Different types of crystal have different shapes and colors. A particular crystal shape is caused by the variation in the angles of intersection of the plane faces; the color reflects the nature of the materials used in the crystal's formation. Crystals come in many varied forms, from ice to diamonds, from salt to sugar, and from sulphur to quartz. All have their part to play and their place in the natural world.

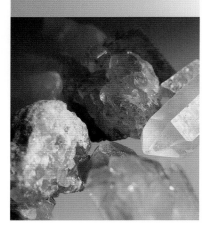

Energy is described as that which gives matter or radiation the ability to do work. There are many forms of energy, including potential (the energy an object has by virtue of its position) and kinetic (the energy of motion). There is also heat energy and electrical energy, for example.

One of the reasons it is so difficult to understand fully the healing power of such things as crystals and magnets is that the energy they give out has no effect whatsoever on any of our senses. We cannot see it, feel it, taste it, or hear it. Magnetic energy is easier to detect than the vibrational energy of a crystal, but special equipment is still necessary for its detection. However, both crystals and magnets have energy that can do work, and this work can be healing.

CRYSTALS

Crystals, like magnets, have the ability to give out energy without loss from the source. As in the case of magnets, the energy vibrations of crystals have been used for healing since before records began. It is said that the lost kingdom of Atlantis used crystal power to provide most of its energy needs. Today, the accuracy of the quartz watch is based on the steady and unchanging vibrational frequency of specific types of quartz crystals.

The power of the crystal's vibration has always been with us but we seem to have lost the ability to detect, respond, and use the powers of the earth's natural crystals. We now make so many artificial crystals that we seem to have destroyed our connection to the natural ones.

NATURAL VIBRATIONS

There are many other natural sources of vibrational energy, for example ley lines, which may be magnetic in origin. The healing power of a tree and the vibration level of a homeopathic remedy are both examples of vibrational benefactors. The peacefulness of a garden, the tranquil nature of old woodland, the sheer beauty of a rose are all vibrational effects. When we are young we have a vibrational frequency that is more in tune with frantic activity, and as we get older we automatically retune to a slower, more gentle frequency. We change, so it follows that the things with which we are in tune also change.

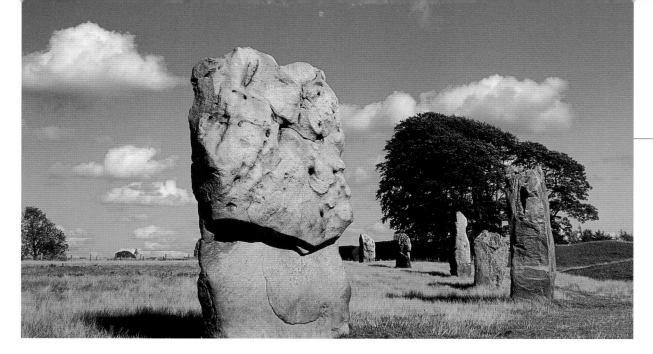

Quantum physics has shown us that vibration is at the heart of all that we call matter. Chaos theory has taught us that the smallest event can have significant and far-reaching consequences. A large mass of energy may need only the slightest vibrational energy to set it free. When faced with this knowledge, the natural vibrational forces of crystals and magnets take on a new significance.

VIBRATIONAL ENERGY AND WAVE FORMS

Energy that is given off in bursts can be described as vibrating, and energy that fluctuates in intensity but is consistently present can be said to be a wave form. When we detect only the peaks of a fluctuating wave of energy, we can be fooled into believing it is vibrational. When two wave forms of similar energy are tuned so that the peaks coincide, the strength of that energy is added together. When they are tuned so that the peak of one is coincidental with the trough of the other, the total energy is diminished. If the waves are of two different and incompatible types of energy, they will simply coexist and not affect each other. Using energy patterns to counteract unwanted energy patterns in the body, or to enhance desirable energy patterns, may be the key to long-term future healthcare.

Modern electromagnetic devices are tuned to give off a particular wave form of energy or are programmed to vary—within controlled limits—the energy wave forms they do give off. Research is being carried out into the fact that the wave form of a person's electrical (brain) activity can be calmed or enhanced either by being in the field of a counterbalancing wave form or in the field of a wave form that enhances the natural one. Another theory is that if an electrical impulse from a human is slightly off its optimum output, then the addition of "wrong" pulses of energy can cause the body to correct the error that was originally present and therefore rebalance the whole system.

It has been suggested that magnetism was used to move huge stones, like these at Avebury stone circle, England.

ENERGY CAUSES CHANGE

If we look at the effect of applying energy to just about anything, we see that it causes changes to occur. If you have difficulty imagining something as small as an atom, think bigger. In pool the game starts with a group of balls organized into a triangular shape. Energy is applied by sending another ball into this organized shape. The result is a relatively random repositioning. The same thing happens when energy is applied to an atom: one of the electrons, which was previously in its proper position, is pushed out and the new shape is random. The difference between charged atoms and a pool table is that the charged atoms will try to correct themselves. The consternation caused if the balls on a pool table tried to reset themselves would be wonderful to see!

Electromagnetism and healing

The most common form of electromagnetic equipment we have in our homes is the speakers in radios, television sets, and telephones. In these devices, sound waves are transformed into electrical impulses and conducted along wires that are wrapped around the metal base of the speaker; this base is attached to a tight diaphragm. The electrical pulse causes a temporary magnetic field to be set up, and this moves the metal base, which moves the diaphragm, and releases it again. The movement of the diaphragm disturbs the air and creates a sound wave that replicates the one that caused the electrical impulse. The creation of the electrical impulse is the reverse of this; sound waves move a diaphragm, which moves a metal bar wrapped with a coil of wire, creating an electrical impulse in the wire.

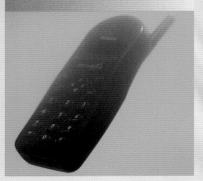

Electromagnetic devices use electrically generated magnetic fields to achieve improvements in well-being. They differ from permanent magnets in that the magnetic field (energy) is not constant; instead it is given out in pulses or in a wave of undulating strength. There is scientific evidence of the beneficial effects of micromagnetic waves in maintaining health. For example, astronauts on early space flights suffered from so-called space sickness when traveling too far from the earth's magnetic field, but the problem was solved by the development of equipment to replicate these signals. Studies suggest that the body responds to micromagnetic waves by increasing the brain's output of the pain inhibitors endorphins, and also by reducing those hormones that increase our stress levels.

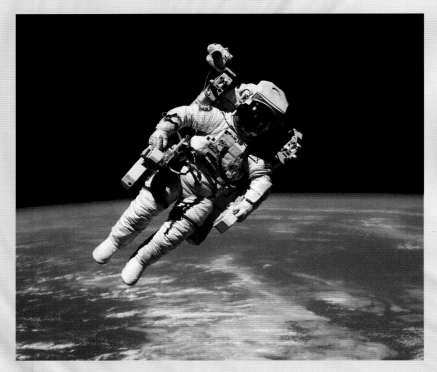

The manipulation of micromagnetic waves helped early astronauts combat space sickness.

PULSED MAGNETIC FIELD GENERATORS

Pulsed magnetic field generators (PMFGs) have been around for about twenty years. Devices such as the Biotron evolved into the Novagen, then the Medigen, all the time becoming smaller, lighter, and more user-friendly. These devices give out a series of magnetic energy pulses from a battery-powered coil of wire. The pulse is a fixed wave form and is always steady. In the more sophisticated equipment, the pulsed micromagnetic field is tuned to the wave patterns of the animal involved, including the human animal, and can be used to affect the energy impulses that the patient gives out. These devices are small and light—0.7 ounces (19 g)—and battery powered to provide a varying magnetic field of up to 200 micro-tesla (2,000 gauss). The time between peaks of magnetic energy is tuned to match the wave patterns in the brain of the subject. A further refinement is the Empulse device, in which the timing of the peaks of energy output is tuned to fit exactly the wave pattern of each specific wearer. The Empulse equipment is intended to work directly on brain patterns, to treat such complaints as migraine and multiple sclerosis. The very latest devices such as the Aegis are programed to produce differing vibrational patterns over a 28-day cycle (the natural cycle of the earth and all things living on it).

The Medicur, another extremely low-frequency radiation device, works in a similar way but is intended to be used for short periods—ten minutes, three times a day—and has a peak energy output of 500 micro-tesla (5,000 gauss). Because the Medicur works directly on damaged tissue rather than on brain waves, it is placed on an area of injury.

GEOPATHIC STRESS NEUTRALIZERS

There are also electromagnetic devices to counter the distortions caused by household equipment, such as electrical cables, televisions, microwave ovens, computers, etc, which set up magnetic fields that are not natural to our environment. Geopathic stress neutralizers are designed to reduce the stress caused by the distorted magnetic fields that occur in modern homes. Any equipment to neutralize these distortions should help to keep us calm and healthy, and improve our efficiency.

BIG MAGNETS

Huge electromagnets, used in such places as foundries and junk-metal yards, have the power to lift tons of metal and release them again at the flick of a switch. Turning off the electrical current means the lifting part of the machine is no longer a magnet, so the load is released.

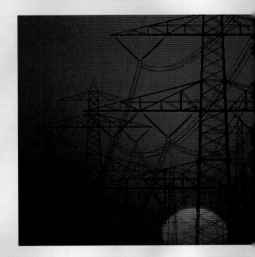

Living or working near power cables can have an effect on our health—and it's not always noticeable. If you are feeling tired or ill, you may be feeling the affects of distorted magnetic fields in your home.

Healing with subtle vibrational energy

Everything gives off vibrations, or put another way, everything, from an individual's aura to a pure crystal, emanates energy. It is easier to consider this as a vibration rather than waves of energy, but these are merely different names for the same thing. An aura may have a complex vibration with harmonics (these are when a wave form interacts with another wave form; the combination sets up both a total [combined] wave form and a regular variation), which would show up as steps, or kinks, in a graph, with mini-peaks and undulations leading up to the main peak of activity. An electromagnetic device can be made with a simple wave form that does not have harmonics, or with complex and variable frequencies to match those in the individual body. These machines use vibrational frequencies between 0.5 Hz and 25.5 Hz. (The Hz is the number of peaks of vibration per second; 1 Hz equals 60 peaks of vibration per minute.) The frequencies used in electromagnetic therapy range from 4.1 Hz to treat migraine to 13 Hz to treat arthritis. Just as with most forms of natural medicine, a particular vibrational frequency will affect different people in different ways. Applying a set frequency to different harmonic combinations gives different results.

The first problem is to identify the vibrational makeup of each individual. Every event in our lives leaves a "footprint," which becomes part of our total makeup. In

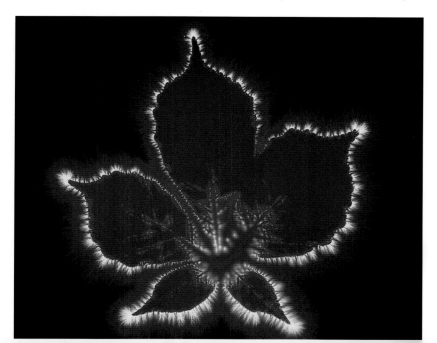

Energy is given off by every living thing, and a Kirlian photograph can capture that on film. Here a chestnut leaf emanates a stunning purple and white light.

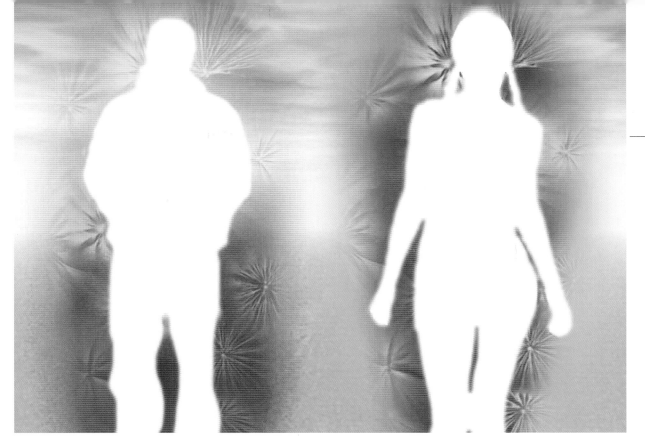

other words, every event changes the harmonics of our subtle energy. The past changes the harmonics of our internal subtle energy, while the future—our fears and anticipations—affects the external energy—the aura.

The objective of magnetic and electromagnetic therapy is to increase the subject's resilience over a period of time. It cannot prevent negative thoughts or the invasion of a virus, but it can make the subtle energy stronger and more stable so that there is more resistance to setbacks and therefore a faster recovery. In electromagnetic devices, the correcting vibrations are produced by a small battery powering a tiny electromagnet. When the battery is switched on, an electromagnetic field is produced. The duration of time that the battery is switched on and the frequency of that switching on are what causes the variation in vibrational frequency. The switch is off for much longer (relatively, and we are talking tiny fractions of a second) than it is on, thereby ensuring a long battery life.

The aura is a complex, energetic entity, which vibrates at a very high level. Fears, hopes, and anticipations can affect this external energy, sometimes resulting in color changes within the aura.

COMPLEMENTARY TREATMENTS

Throughout history, vibrational devices, especially crystals, have been used for healing. Experience has shown that vibrational and magnetic treatments enhance and improve whatever other form of treatment is being offered. A magnet therapist's objective is to improve the total well-being of the patient as quickly and effectively as possible, so they will usually encourage the use of additional and enhancing complementary treatments.

The healing power of electromagnetism

Although static or electromagnetic fields have been used for many centuries to control pain and other medical problems, there has been no scientific research into their effectiveness until recently. But the positive results of such research suggest that magnet therapy could play an important role in conventional medicine and rehabilitation. Electromagnetic field studies show promise in the treatment of bone and neurological pain, and sleep disorders. However, caution is needed in

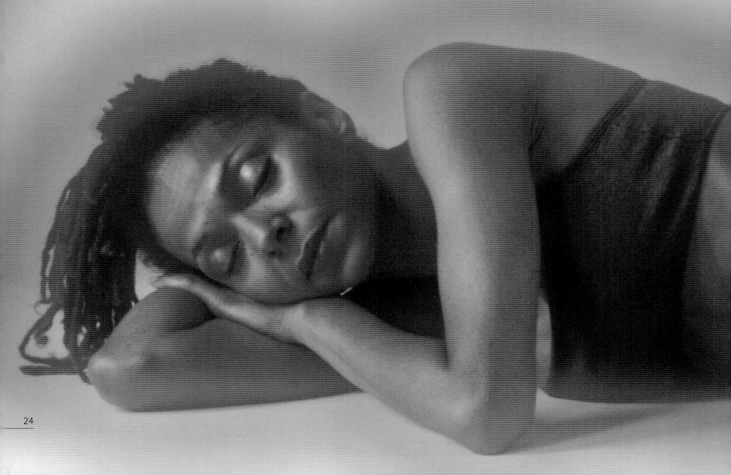

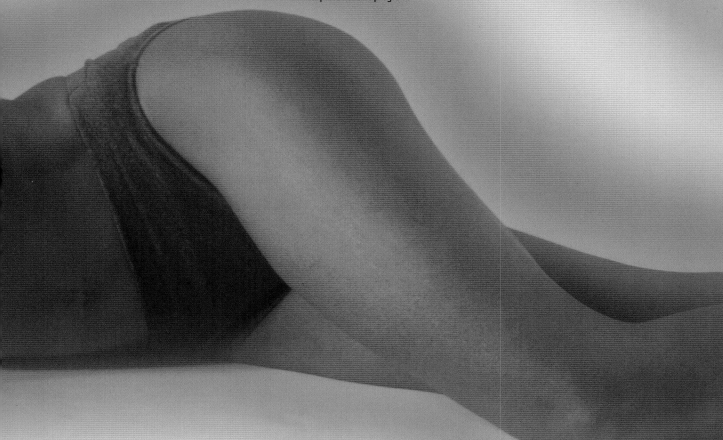

evaluating nonscientifically-based claims about curing diseases, such as those found on several websites on the Internet. Pulsating electromagnetic fields (PEMFs) have been used as therapeutic modalities for at least forty years. A well recognized and standard use of PEMFs is an enhancement of the rate of healing of nonunion fractures, and recent research has reported good results in using PEMFs to treat migraine headaches and manage multiple sclerosis.

The therapeutic use of electromagnetism means that it could play an important part in the healthcare of the future. With other alternative therapies, electromagnetism could combine with conventional medicine to provide a complete holistic program.

✳ Magnets and plant growth

SEED EXPERIMENTS

Some seeds were planted with their points facing north, some with them pointing south, and others at random. The seeds pointing north and south sprouted earlier than those planted at random.

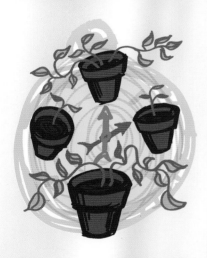

Magnets can affect seed growth, and can speed up sprouting times.

Over the centuries there have been countless experiments to show the effect of magnets on plant growth. The magnets cause plant molecules to align relative to each other, which in turn improves the flow of nutrients around the plants and increases growth rates. Louis Pasteur (1822–95) is allegedly the first person to note the positive effects on plant growth of the earth's own magnetic field.

It has been discovered that plants kept within the magnetic field grow faster and produce more vegetation and fruit. Russian studies have shown that plants irrigated with magnetized water were found to have grown 20 to 40 percent faster than the control plants. Even almost-dead plants have been revived when exposed to a magnetic field or given magnetized water.

As mentioned previously, water that has been subjected to a magnetic field has a reduced surface tension, which enables it to pass more easily through the cell membranes than normal water. This may explain why plants do better when given magnetized water. Surface tension holds the molecules of water together on an exposed surface, stopping them from entering another substance; surface resistance is the ability to prevent other substances from entering the water.

THE ARNDT-SCHULE LAW

During many of the plant and animal experiments, what is known as the Arndt-Schule law was seen to apply. This law states that weak stimulants encourage life activity, middle stimulants tend to hold back life activity, and strong stimulants can stop or destroy life activity. Something called the "inverse square rule" also applies to magnets. This means that the strength of the magnetic field gets weaker very quickly as we move away from the magnet. Generally, it is said that a 6,000-gauss magnet produces a middle stimulant, but this would only apply at the surface of the magnet; the effect even a few millimeters into the body will be a weak to middle stimulation.

PLANT EXPERIMENTS

In plant trials, seeds that had been exposed to a magnetic field sprouted more quickly and had deeper and broader roots than untreated seeds. Plants given water magnetized by direct contact with a north-seeking pole grew long and thin, but plants given water magnetized by contact with a south-seeking pole grew short and thick. Other experiments indicate that magnetism has a positive effect on the enzyme processes in plants. Russian farmers have been able to improve the size of tomatoes and eggplants using this information.

Cooked food has been shown to stay fresh longer under the influence of a north-seeking pole than under the influence of a south-seeking pole. It seems that a north-seeking pole slows down fermentation, while a south-seeking pole speeds it up. (Food mats containing north-seeking magnets, which can help food stay fresher for longer, can be purchased for this particular purpose.)

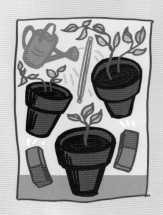

EXPERIMENTS TO TRY AT HOME

It is possible to do your own experiments at home. Fill three pots with the same potting soil and sprinkle the same number of mustard seeds into each pot. Place a magnet under two of the pots. Under one, have the north-seeking pole facing upward, under the other, have the south-seeking pole facing upward. The third pot has no magnets. Keep the light conditions and temperature the same for all three pots. Give each pot the same amount of water at the same time each day and observe which seeds sprout first and which grow most quickly.

You could introduce other variables into your plant experiments. Prepare another three pots as in the previous experiments, but use water that has stood in a glass jar on top of a magnet for 24 hours. Compare the growth of these seeds with those that have been given ordinary water. Try these experiments using different-strength magnets. Make sure that you keep all other factors the same except for the magnet strength.

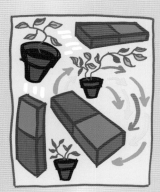

Conducting plant experiments with magnets and magnetized water can show exactly how magnetism can improve fertility and growth. A small-scale trial could change the way you grow fruit and vegetables forever!

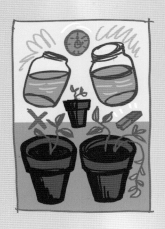

✳ | Magnets and fluid flows

Water becomes ionized when it flows through the metal pipes that transport it. Magnets can change the arrangement of ions in the water, stabilizing the atoms and changing the electrical charges of the molecules.

WATER

Water that flows through pipes often contains deposits such as sodium, potassium, calcium, and lime. These deposits can get stuck to the sides of the pipes, causing obstructions. Magnetized water used in a closed pipe system does not leave a residue in the pipes, and in some experiments it has been shown that magnetized water will actually help remove mineral deposits.

Both magnetic fields and electrical currents can cause ionization of water. An ion is an electrically charged atom, or group of atoms, formed by the loss or gain of one or more electrons. The energy given out by a magnetic field or an electrical current causes the electrons around the atoms to become imbalanced. The atom that is thrown out of balance will seek to stabilize itself by being attracted to whatever has the required polarity, or "charge," necessary to rebalance it: this causes the water to ionize.

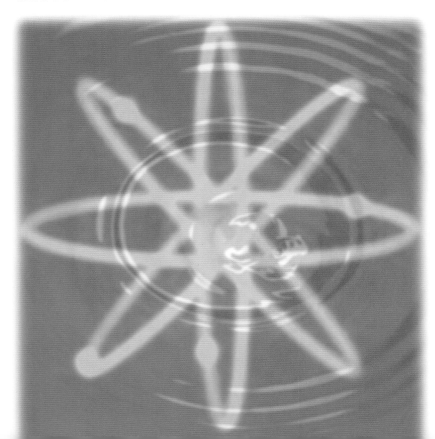

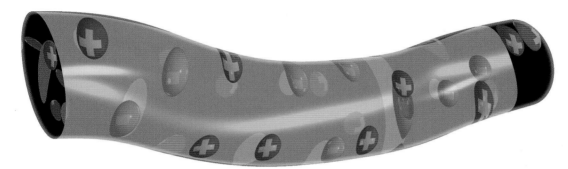

If water can be affected by magnets, then so can blood, which is also a fluid. The application of magnets can line up all the molecules within the blood so it flows more freely, and there is less chance of any damaging deposits being left behind on the walls of the vessel.

As water flows along pipes the friction of the water rubbing on them could cause partial ionization, which in turn will cause the water to deposit some of the chemicals it contains. Water can be softened, i.e. have its minerals removed, by ion exchange, which is a process whereby ions are exchanged between a solution (the water) and a solid: one atom becomes destabilized and seeks something that has the required polarity necessary to rebalance it.

Magnets can also affect the ions in water; they add energy to change the electrical charges of the atoms and molecules that make up the water, and can stabilize the atoms within the liquid too.

BLOOD

The same effect can be seen in other fluids, such as blood. Like water, blood contains various chemical substances and sometimes deposits these on the walls of the blood vessels it flows through, with detrimental effects; this results in clogged-up arteries, raised blood pressure, and thrombosis. If the molecules of the blood are lined up and the electrical charges of those molecules are stable, blood flow will improve and deposits decrease. Magnets can be used to help this process.

ELECTROLYTES

When ions are formed by passing an electrical current through a liquid, that liquid is known as an electrolyte. An electrolyte is able to conduct electricity.

ENERGY FLOWS

Energy itself behaves like a fluid. It travels through the body along energy paths known as meridians. Magnets can influence the flow of this life energy or life force (also known as chi or qi) as it moves around the meridians of the body.

29

✳ | How magnets affect us

MAGNETISM AND PLANET EARTH

The strength of the earth's magnetic field fluctuates year by year. It seems that at the moment the strength is lower than it was 500 years ago. These fluctuations are mainly due to the fact that the earth's magnetic forces are generated by the iron core of the earth rotating on a particular north–south axis. The fact that this iron core and the main body of the earth do not rotate at the same speed causes changes in the surface measurement of the magnetic forces. The effects of these distortions in magnetic energy on humans are almost impossible to quantify: it has been claimed that this causes problems and equally it has been claimed that no adverse effects have been experienced. In fact, these magnetic forces change all the time, and differ from place to place, so we are constantly moving from one level of force to another. Manufactured objects cause localized distortions in the flows of magnetic energy, which have subtle effects on each and every one of us. The largest distortions are caused by the transmission of electrical power. Most industrialized processes that involve magnets, however, are self-contained and do not cause any energy distortions.

Some magnetic fields, such as the ones surrounding the earth, lodestones, and some iron-ore-rich mountains, exist in nature; other magnetic fields are created by the passage of electricity around our homes. The computer, television, radio, telephone, and just about every gadget that uses electricity, particularly if the gadget makes a noise, will have some form of magnet within it. All of these magnetic fields will vary in strength and frequency. According to the "inverse square law," the fields are weak when we are some distance from the source, but they do still have the ability to disturb the natural magnetic fields. Our modern world is constantly permeated by waves of energy that are not natural to the earth—radio, television, mobile phones, microwave ovens, even the sounds from the traffic. These are all waves or constantly varying levels of magnetism.

GEOPATHIC STRESS

When the earth's vibrations rise up through the earth and are distorted by weak electromagnetic fields, created by subterranean running water coupled with

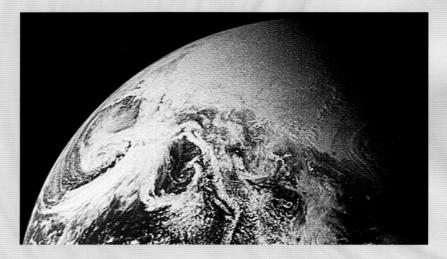

The magnetic field around the earth is never at a constant strength, and fluctuates yearly. It is not known how these changes affect our lives.

certain mineral concentrations, fault lines, and underground cavities, the result is geopathic stress. The vibration distortion can become abnormally high and is harmful to living organisms. If you seem to be always ill, slightly below par, or depressed, perhaps geopathic stress in your home or workplace could be the source of the problem. If these feelings started after moving to a new house or workplace or if you feel better when on vacation or working at another location, if other people in the same house or workplace also suffer the same symptoms, or if the building seems cold and damp even with the heating on, then you may need to try to neutralize the geopathic stress in your living environment.

There are many practices that can help to relieve the negative effects of geopathic stress. The ancient Chinese art of feng shui can enhance the flow of positive energy and free up areas of geopathic stress in your living and work environment. You can purchase geopathic stress neutralizers, which give out frequencies of vibration that attempt to neutralize the distorted ones. Many people use crystals in the same way.

COPING STRATEGIES

Many of us spend far too much time in unnatural, enclosed spaces, such as cars, trains, and underground transportation systems. The frequency of the vibrational energy we are subjected to in these situations may be a contributing factor in the rise of stress-related problems. Since we do not live in an ideal world, we cannot always avoid these vibrational distortions, but we can develop our own individual coping strategies. We are all individuals, each with our own particular vibrational frequency, so there is no universal panacea, no cure that suits all of us. Each one of us must find out, through trial and error, which methods work best for us.

There are many coping strategies that can help us to overcome the adverse effects of vibrations that are out of tune with our individual needs. These include yoga exercises, walks in the fresh air, meditation, and deep breathing, particularly after a lengthy spell confined in a space subjected to unsuitable vibrations. Some coping strategies, such as smoking and drinking alcohol, should be used in small doses only; overuse of an unsuitable coping strategy could become part of the problem rather than the solution.

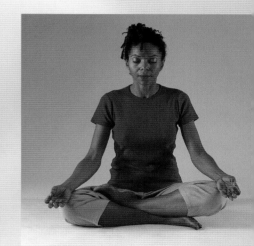

Yoga can help combat the effect of unnatural vibrations. It can also make us more aware of our own vibrational frequency.

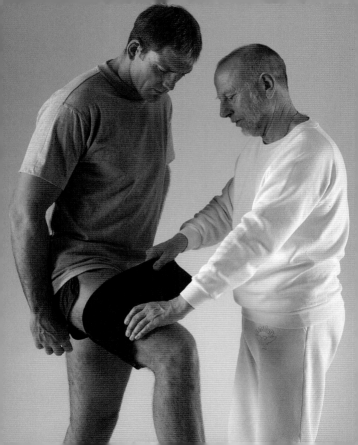

✳ | # Chapter two

Using magnets Constant levels of magnetic energy can also
be used to great effect. These are provided by permanent magnets.
Permanent magnets can be used to improve our individual
well-being and to speed up the natural healing process; they give
out energy at a constant level and rely on energy transmission and
the "lining up" effect that magnetic forces have on substances—they
do not vibrate as electromagnets do. When placed on acupuncture
points, small self-adhesive magnets act as slow-release acupuncture
needles, but a magnet simply can be placed on a painful area to
obtain some relief. Flexible magnetized bandages can also be
wrapped around the site of an injury to relieve pain.

Permanent magnets and healing

Small magnets for use on the skin are usually mounted on an adhesive pad.

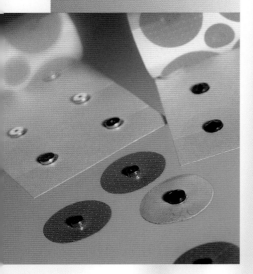

Magnets have a variety of applications. As discussed previously, the controlled variation in the strength of a small magnetic field using electromagnetic devices can have beneficial effects on our health.

PERMANENT MAGNETS

Permanent magnets give out energy at a constant level. They rely on the energy transmission and the organizing, regulating, or "lining up" effect that magnetic forces have on material, rather than the vibrational effects created by electromagnets that switch the energy off and on very quickly.

Permanent magnets are also used to improve our individual well-being and to speed up the natural healing process. Later in this book we will explore, in detail, the use of small permanent magnets placed on the acupuncture points, where they act as slow-release needles. These same small adhesive magnets can be used as purely localized treatments, without prior knowledge of energy meridians.

The small permanent magnets commonly available for self-help are ferrite (iron-based) magnets, which are also known as ceramic magnets, and are usually preset in place on a self-adhesive pad. These usually have the north pole uppermost when you open the package, indicating that it is the north pole that will be in contact with the skin. These can be purchased in a variety of magnetic strengths from 200 to 9,000 gauss. When buying over the counter from a pharmacist, it is not always obvious from the packaging what strength the magnets are or which pole will be in contact with the skin. If in doubt, ask the supplier or producer. However, specialized suppliers and therapists can provide small magnets in different strengths and with clear instructions on which pole touches the skin; some magnets are even reversible so that the therapist can have a choice of poles for each particular application.

MAGNETIC BANDAGES

Magnetic strips or bandages usually contain bonded powdered magnetic iron material in a fabric. These can be preformed to fit around a specific joint such as a knee or elbow. It is possible to buy thumb supports, neck and shoulder wraps, and even headbands with magnetized material in them.

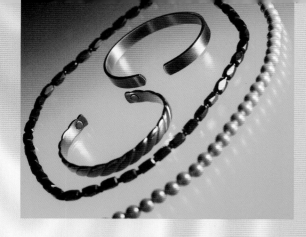

Magnets can also be worn in the form of attractive jewelry, and can influence the whole body.

MAGNETIC JEWELRY

Magnets also come in decorative forms, designed to be worn inconspicuously. Magnetic necklaces, rings, bracelets, and earrings can all be obtained in a huge range of appealing designs. A 1,000-gauss necklace, for example, provides medium magnetic therapy to the neck and shoulders, while a 2,500-gauss bracelet can provide strong magnetic therapy to the whole body. Magnetic jewelry can make the use of magnets much more accessible to the nonspecialist.

FOOT SUPPORTS

Our feet are our main contact with the earth and the main conductor of the earth's energy up into our bodies. They are also a common center for discomfort. There are many designs for shoe inserts—insoles—available, and some of these contain magnets or magnetic strips. It is always worth checking on the condition of the arch of the foot before deciding on magnetic insoles. Arch-correction supports have been known to improve posture, balance, and even migraines. By changing the shape and "attitude" of the foot while in a shoe, these simple devices can have an effect on the whole postural structure of the body and may provide a solution without the need for magnetic energy input. However, a combination of arch correction and magnetic energy may be an enhanced solution to postural problems caused by fallen or partially collapsed arches.

Self-adhesive magnets can be worn unobtrusively and during your daily walk or exercise routine.

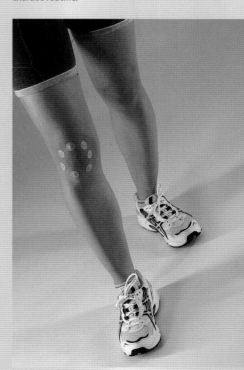

TREATMENT WHILE ASLEEP

There are mattresses, underblankets, pillows, and overlays that incorporate magnets or bonded-in magnetized material. Their magnetic energy can have a therapeutic effect, helping to ease stress and muscular aches while you are sleeping. They can also help insomnia.

OTHER PERMANENT MAGNET DEVICES

Magnetic massage devices, hairbrushes, eye masks, grip-strengthening balls, and wafer-thin magnets to use on the chakras are also available from specialist suppliers and through therapists. All of this equipment can be very useful if it is chosen and used correctly. Consult your therapist if you are at all unsure.

Contraindications and dangers

We are surrounded and constantly bombarded by electromagnetic waves of low-power energy. The variation in their levels, especially when added to the variations that exist from natural sources, makes it impossible to predict accurately the effects of any large-scale additional electromagnetic field. But, in magnet therapy, we are only dealing with small-scale and locally applied fields. The electromagnetic vibration of wave-form devices is intended to correct the effects of the bombardment by the energy waves from non-natural sources. Magnet therapy is safe and will help relieve pain, improve well-being, and speed recovery, but you must take care to ensure that you act responsibly toward your body.

The following is a list of precautions regarding the use of magnets and electromagnetic equipment:

• *Do not use magnets if you have a pacemaker or any other mechanical or electromechanical equipment implanted within your body.*

• *Do not bring blood to a freshly torn muscle that is still bleeding internally. Massage and magnets should not be applied to such areas for several days after the injury: three to five days is usually long enough, but if the tear is severe, or the patient is slow-healing, then it could take up to ten to fourteen days. In such a severe case, however, medical assistance is vital.*

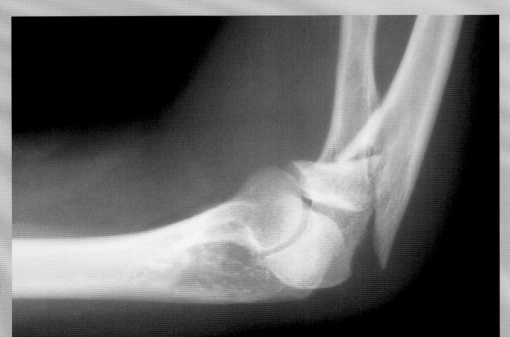

Care must be taken when using magnets on a broken limb. It is imperative to wait until any internal bleeding has stopped before commencing treatment.

- *During pregnancy, do not use powerful magnets in the abdominal area because the effects on the baby and its surrounding fluids are unknown and therefore unpredictable. Magnets worn on point P6 (the wrist) for nausea should be safe.*
- *Do not use magnets on open wounds.*
- *Do not use magnets taken from old electrical equipment—the strength of magnets used in old-fashioned loudspeakers can be too powerful.*
- *Do not go near powerful transmitters of any sort of magnetic, radio, vibrational, or wave-form energy. The dangers of X-ray and gamma-ray transmitters are well known, but some of the dangers of high-power radio transmitters are less so.*

Human beings are very complex. The physical body, the mind, the emotions, and the ethereal (spiritual) body are codependent realms that make up a human being, and each is affected by what is happening in the other realms. So it follows that magnetic forces can affect the total human being at the physical, mental, emotional, and spiritual levels.

The complete interconnection that exists between so many different parts of the whole means that even a pain in the right big toe may have a relevance to the heart or some other vital organ. There is no need to be frightened of every ache and pain, but there is a need to take care of your body and ensure that a life-threatening condition does not go untreated because its seriousness was not recognized. Remember to consult your medical practitioner in all cases of ill-health. Diagnosis of the cause of any particular symptom requires a great deal of training, experience, and knowledge, and still it is possible to get it wrong. Guessing without adequate knowledge is very dangerous. Your intuition is a great guiding force but it should be backed up with reliable information.

CANCER AND MAGNETS

The fact that magnets improve the flow of blood and lymph fluids does cause concern for many people when dealing with cancer. They fear that by stimulating the blood flow and lymphatic system, cancer cells can be transported around the body. But blood and lymph fluids are constantly flowing through the body, even without stimulation. Other stimulation techniques such as massage have been shown to improve patients' well-being, so magnets could also be beneficial.

POWER TRANSMISSION LINES

A great deal of research evidence indicates that high-voltage power transmission lines are safe; at the same time, there is opposing evidence, showing potential dangers. In light of these conflicting opinions it is best to be cautious and try to avoid being near transmission lines whenever possible.

The body's transportation systems

The human body is a wonderful piece of plumbing. The pipework system of the blood vessels alone would have the average heating engineer lost in admiration. Add in the capillaries, the lymph system, the pulmonary network, and the urinary pipework and this admiration turns into sheer wonderment.

We have already looked at the effect magnetic forces have on fluid flows in pipes, so the effect of carefully placed magnets on the transportation systems of the body should be easy to visualize. The blood vessels, blood, and other pipework systems that make up the transport infrastructure of the body carry nutrients, blood, enzymes, and hormones to wherever they are needed and then cart away waste byproducts, ready for filtration, storage, and ejection from the body.

THE RESPIRATORY SYSTEM

When we breathe in, we transport a complex collection of gases to the lungs. In the lungs, these gases are separated and the required elements absorbed into the blood. The unwanted elements are then breathed back out into the environment, where they complete their natural cycle and eventually end up as useful air again. Such a smooth transition, from one part of the transportation system to another, is part of the wonder of being human.

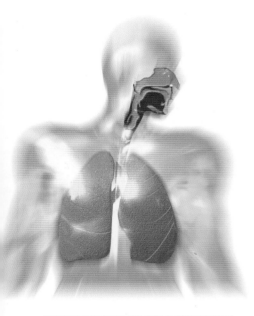

FLUID IN THE BODY

The average body is roughly 66 percent water. The amount of water and the fact that the transportation system is made up of fluids flowing though pipes explains why magnets can have such an effect on the human body.

The respiratory system (see left) comes into its own during any kind of exercise. The fitter you are, the more efficient it is.

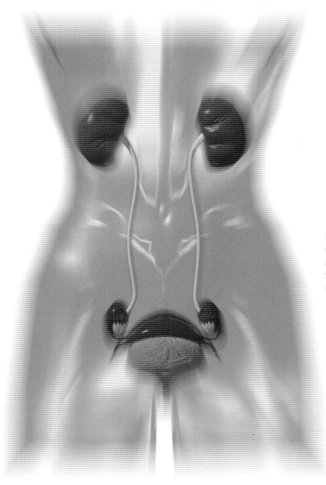

Magnets can help the smooth running of another fluid flow—that to be found in the urinary system.

BLOOD VESSELS

Once the blood has passed though the lungs, it is conducted, via pulmonary veins, into the heart. The heart is a muscular pump that creates sufficient pressure to push the blood around the rest of the system. Blood flows away from the heart in blood vessels called arteries. Blood returns to the heart in blood vessels called veins. Arteries carry oxygenated and outgoing blood; veins carry returning, deoxygenated blood that contains the unwanted byproducts of our activities.

THE URINARY SYSTEM

The urinary system is another collection of pipes conveying fluids through the body. Liquid waste, produced as the byproducts of activity, is expelled from the body as sweat or as urine. The name urine comes from the fact that it is made up of a mixture of water and urea. Urea is poisonous and is taken out of the body through the liver. The blood carries the urea from the liver to the kidneys, which filter it out of the blood and combine it with water to make urine. Urine travels along yet more tubes into the bladder, and when a sufficient quantity collects in the bladder, it is expelled out of the body. Magnetic forces can smooth the flows in this transportation system as well.

FACTS ABOUT BLOOD

Blood is pumped into the arteries about 70 times a minute. The pressure travels along the arteries like a wave. This wave is the pulse, and the amount of pressure required to stop blood from flowing is the higher figure shown when blood pressure is taken.

There are about 62,000 miles (100,000 km) of blood vessels in the average adult human body. The blood vessels are quite large when they are leaving, or just returning to, the heart, but they get smaller and smaller as they find their way around the body until they form the smallest tubes, called capillaries. These can be so small that they have a wall thickness that is a single cell only. It is here that most of the delivery of the required oxygen and chemicals and the collection of unwanted byproducts takes place. As the blood returns along its path, now carrying the waste byproducts, the tubes become thicker and are joined by inputs from other capillaries as they flow back to the heart.

The average adult body holds about 6–7 quarts (5–6 liters) of blood. The red blood cells, which give blood its color, carry the oxygen. These red blood cells have a useful life of around four months and travel about 932 miles (1,500 km) in that time.

✳ | Skin—the surface layer

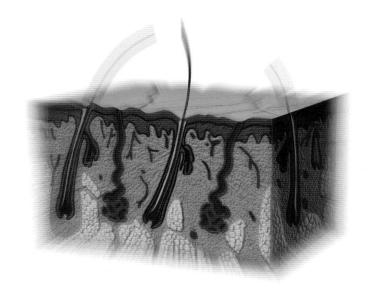

Magnets can improve blood flow to the skin and surrounding area, bringing healing enzymes quickly to the site of an injury.

The skin is where we apply magnetic influences, so it is important to know what skin is and what it does.

Skin is relatively elastic and holds the flesh together while protecting us from harmful substances, such as dirt, which would otherwise get into the flesh. Skin thickness varies, depending on which part of the body it covers; skin generally is about ¹⁄₁₆ in (2 mm) thick, but on the soles of the feet it is more than ²⁄₁₆ in (4 mm) thick and on the eyelids it is ¹⁄₄₈ in (0.5 mm).

Skin is made up of layers. The outer layer is called the epidermis and is mainly dead cells that contain keratin, which help make the skin waterproof and resistant. This layer is in a state of constant change; as it is worn away, it is replaced by new cells from below. Under the epidermis is a thicker and more elastic layer called the dermis. In this layer there are glands that provide the oil that helps keep the skin soft and supple, and various types of nerve endings that enable us to sense pain, touch, and temperature. Sensitivity to touch is governed by the number of tactile nerve endings there are in the skin; hands and lips have more nerve endings than the rest of the body and so are much more sensitive. Tiny capillary blood vessels are also in the dermis. Blood vessels close to the outer edge of our skin play a vital role in the control of body temperature. When we are too hot, they widen to allow more blood to the surface to cool us off; when we are cold, they close up to preserve the blood at a deeper level. Under the dermis level of the skin is a layer of fat that stores chemical energy.

The nervous system

Nerves are the communication network, carrying messages throughout the body. The working parts of the nervous system are millions of interconnected nerve cells called neurones. They pick up signals in one part of the nervous system and send them to another, where they may be relayed to other neurones, or bring about some action (such as contraction of muscle fibers). Neurones are divided into three types, according to their function: sensory neurones, which convey information from the body's sense organs to the central nervous system; integrative neurones, which process the information received; and motor neurones, which initiate voluntary and involuntary actions. The brain acts as a control center, sorting information and deciding on physical responses. The information from sight, touch, hearing, taste, and smell is all gathered and collated for comparison with previous events and known facts. The body responds to these stimuli in various ways, and because the past experiences of two people may differ, their responses will also differ. The sight of a dog may cause one person to recoil in fear, while another may welcome it. (In ordinary, everyday language there is a tendency to confuse the emotional responses with the nervous ones. We often talk about someone being nervous when the person is actually suffering from anxiety or some other form of emotional ill-health.)

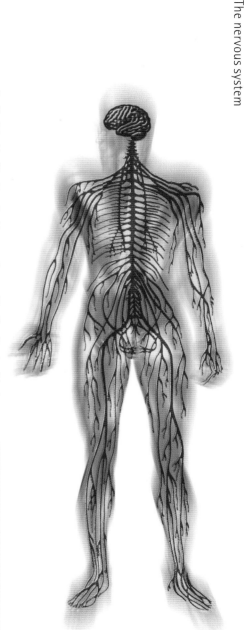

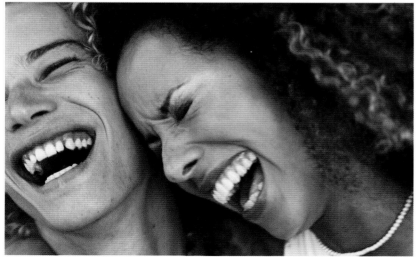

Laughing with friends can relax the body and mind, helping to soothe the nervous system (see above).

✳ | The digestive system

Digestion is the process that breaks down food into substances that can be absorbed and used by the body for energy, growth, and repair. The whole system is one continuous muscular tube, about 33 ft (10 m) in length, with various connections and holding stations along the way. This alimentary canal starts at the mouth and ends at the anus.

Digestion starts in the mouth where food is partially broken down and the absorption process begins. The salivary glands produce excretions that contain enzymes; these start the chemical process of breaking down the food we have eaten. The chewed-up food passes down the esophagus into the stomach, where, under normal conditions, it will stay for about four hours. Here it is broken down by the action of various chemicals, mainly acids, that the body produces.

The stomach is a muscular sac and its size and shape varies with its muscular strength and the amount that has been eaten. It has two curvatures, called the greater and the lesser, and is split up into three distinct parts, the cardiac sphincter, the main body of the stomach, and the pyloric sphincter. The entrance to and the

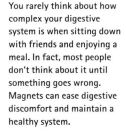

You rarely think about how complex your digestive system is when sitting down with friends and enjoying a meal. In fact, most people don't think about it until something goes wrong. Magnets can ease digestive discomfort and maintain a healthy system.

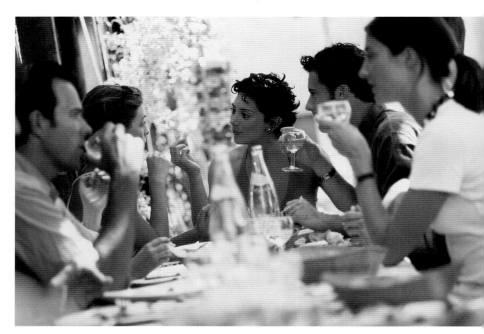

exit from the stomach are via two circular bands of muscle that act as one-way valves: these are the cardiac and the pyloric sphincters. The stomach wall itself has three layers, or membranes, which are arranged in folds; these disappear when the stomach is full or extended. These contain glands that produce the gastric juices, which include the enzymes pepsin and gastrin, as well as hydrochloric acid. The liver, gall bladder, and pancreas all play their parts in the production and storage of these digestive juices. The liver has other functions but the production of digestive bile is one important aspect of its work.

The broken-down food is now transferred to the small intestine, via the duodenal tract—which is where most ulcers occur—through a couple of one-way valves. In the small intestine, much of the nutrient transfer into the blood takes place. Like the stomach, the walls of the small intestine are composed of folded mucus membrane but, unlike the stomach, these folds do not disappear when the small intestine is full. These walls are covered in tiny, fingerlike projections known as villi (villus in the singular) and within these walls are glands that secrete enzymes able to break down proteins and sugars and make them into the chemical constituents needed by the body. The required material passes through the wall of the small intestine into the blood vessels that are attached. This food absorbed by the blood then drains into the liver for processing before it goes into the rest of the body. This process within the small intestine normally takes between 4 and 5 hours to complete. The remaining material then passes into the large intestine, which separates out the water, before it is passed as solid matter into the rectum and so into the anus, where it is stored before it is time for its discharge.

This whole process of digestion can take an astonishing 38 hours—in fact, it is calculated that it normally takes between 27 and 38.5 hours for the food that we place in our mouths eventually to be discharged as waste matter.

HOW MAGNET THERAPY CAN HELP DIGESTION

Magnet therapy can help the digestive system by causing the digestive fluids to align themselves correctly and therefore flow more efficiently through the stomach and intestine. Magnets can also improve the digestion of food by speeding these fluids up and making them work more quickly.

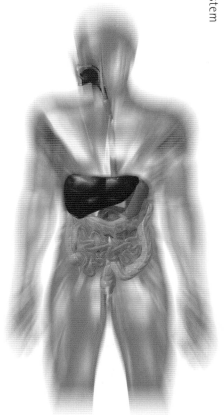

Although complex and lengthy, the digestive system can be helped by the application of magnets. Food absorption and digestion can be improved, easing heartburn and indigestion.

✳ | The pulmonary system

Oxygen fuels all activity, and inefficient oxygen absorption can affect our energy levels. Magnet therapy can improve the function of the lungs, and the flow of air through them.

The pulmonary system provides the body with the oxygen, and some other gases, that are needed to live. The average adult breathes in and out 24,021 pints (13,650 liters) of air in a day. Just as a fire will not burn without oxygen, our bodies will not function unless we have sufficient oxygen in the blood to fuel both brain and muscular activity. The blood uses the chemical iron as part of its way of fixing the gas oxygen so that it can be carried safely within itself. Anemia is a reduction in the quality of the oxygen-carrying pigment hemoglobin in the blood. Because there is not enough capacity to carry oxygen, the body is kept short of one of the most vital components that it needs. The main symptoms are excessive tiredness and fatigue, breathlessness on exertion, pallor, and diminished resistance to infection.

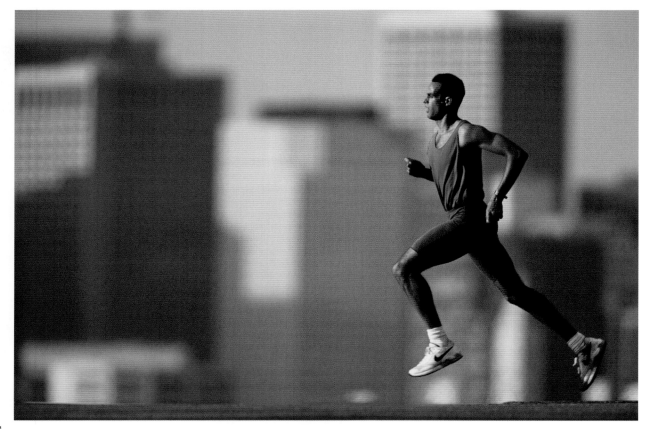

In order to get oxygen to the blood, we first have to breathe it in. The air is filtered and conducted through a series of tubes that get smaller and smaller until they reach the lungs; here a chemical interchange takes place. This is when oxygen is swapped for unwanted byproduct gases such as carbon dioxide. These byproduct gases are then exhaled from the body. Breathing in is called inhalation while breathing out is called exhalation.

The process of respiration starts with the nose. This is part of the upper respiratory tract, which also includes the mouth, the throat, and the sinus cavities. The lower respiratory tract includes the trachea (windpipe), the bronchi, and the lungs. The lungs are not muscular in the way that, for example, the heart is; they do not "work" for themselves. They are inert organs that are pumped by the movement of the diaphragm and the rib cage.

The pulmonary system takes in the air that we breathe, filters out unwanted particles, then carries the cleaner, but still complex, collection of gases into the blood. The unwanted parts are then piped back out into the environment, where they complete their natural cycle and eventually end up as useful air again. Pollution, however, has an effect on our ability to breathe. If there is too much dust in the air then the filter system becomes blocked. Unnaturally fine particles, such as the fibers from some types of asbestos, can evade the filter system and lodge themselves in the lungs, with devastating consequences. Every part of the respiratory system is incredibly delicate in some ways yet remarkably robust in others—we can hold our breath for up to three minutes without harm; we can recover from breathing in harmful gases in a very short time; we can live in cities that have high levels of pollution—but if this system sinks below the minimum needs of the body, then the whole thing can fail.

HOW MAGNET THERAPY CAN
HELP THE PULMONARY SYSTEM

Magnet therapy can help the pulmonary system by relaxing the muscles around the bronchial tubes when they are in spasm, thereby improving the air flow into the lungs. This can be useful for sportspeople, who wish to improve the efficiency of their pulmonary systems, or those suffering from chest infections or asthma.

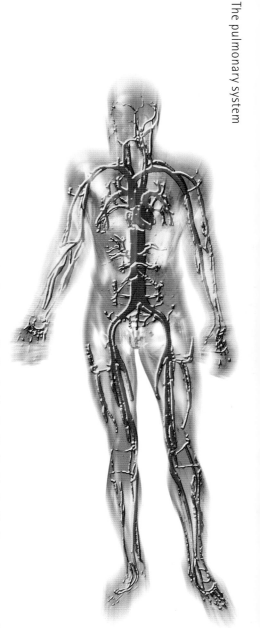

The pulmonary system is extremely resilient. Magnet therapy can help improve the flow of oxygen.

✳ | The skeleton and muscles

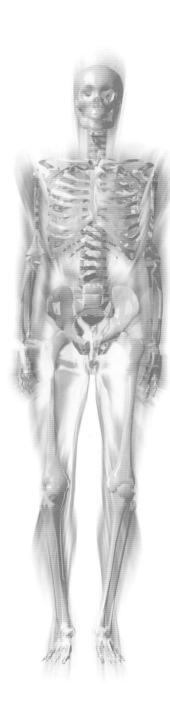

THE SKELETON

It is generally agreed that the human skeleton has 206 bones in it. (There is some disagreement, however, in different textbooks; some take this number to be the number of bones at birth before certain structures fuse together to form what would be one bone in adulthood.) The skeleton has many important functions. It protects soft organs; the skull protects the brain, the ribs protect the lungs, and the spine protects the spinal cord. The skeletal structure also enables us to move freely and the way it interacts with the muscles gives us our posture and shape. The spine, for example, combines with some very strong muscles to hold us upright.

Bones cannot bend very far but movement is made possible by the arrangement of the joints—these can be rigid and fixed (like the plates that form the skull), hinged (like a knee or elbow), ball and socket (as in the arm and shoulders), or gliding joints (as in the spine or wrist). The knee joint is the only joint in the body that is capable of full-hinge articulation: if it was not for the patella (kneecap), the bones would be capable of moving in either a forward or backward direction—just think of a flamingo to get an idea of this!

Joints that allow movement of one bone relative to another have a membrane of cartilage and a sac of lubricating (synovial) fluid between them. This is to stop the bones from rubbing on each other and wearing away. The synovial fluid is white-ish in color and similiar to raw egg white in consistency. Like oil in a machine, it prevents friction between two moving parts. Joints also possess small sacs containing a clear viscous fluid; these are called mucus bursae and act rather like water-filled cushions, absorbing the pressure of movement. For example, there are two of these bursae in the knee joint which act as shock absorbers for the kneecap. If the synovial membrane in a joint becomes inflamed, this is called synovitis—tennis elbow being a common, and painful, example. Bursitis is when the bursae sac becomes inflamed—housemaid's knee is a well-known example of

The skeleton is the framework that keeps us upright and supports all our internal organs. Problems may occur when parts of this structure break, fracture, or deteriorate.

this. Arthritic pain usually affects one or more of the skeletal joints. It has a variety of causes, and some types of arthritic pain can be relieved by magnet therapy. If the cause of the pain is a sluggish flow of synovial fluid, a magnet's ability to improve fluid flows will help.

Bones are very hard and do not take sudden impact well. If a bone is bent beyond the small amount of flexibility it does have then a fracture will occur. If the impact is so great that the covering flesh cannot cushion the blow, then the bone will break. Fractured or broken bones need to be set or repositioned so that the broken parts are in the correct position relative to each other, and then held in this position until the bones mend. Once any internal bleeding has stopped, magnets can help the flow of repair materials to the site of the break or fracture and speed up the mending process.

MUSCLES

A muscle moves a bone in the skeleton by pulling it; the pulling motion is caused by the contraction of the muscle. But muscles can only pull—they cannot push—so every action in the body involves two sets of muscles: one pulls the joint/limb in one direction, and the others pull it back again. Muscles can be overworked, or strained, and damaged by twisting and overstretching, or sprained. These types of injuries will benefit from alternating hot and cold applications and from the use of magnets. Torn muscles are far more serious. In this case the structure of the muscle is ripped apart and there can be internal bleeding. Magnets should not be applied until the internal bleeding has stopped and there is a need to improve blood flow into and around the muscle for healing purposes.

Muscles come in all sorts of shapes and sizes. Some, such as the heart, are constantly working; others have periods of inactivity. Some are small, and others large and powerful. Muscles are made up of rows of fibers, which slide over each other to allow the contractions that provide movement. Muscles are very tough, and it takes a severe injury for a muscle to get torn. The junctions of muscles with bones are generally the most vulnerable areas. Ligaments—bands of tough, fibrous tissue that bind bones together—and cartilage—tough, flexible tissue attached to bones—are often damaged or injured. Magnet therapy can reduce recovery time.

A WORD OF WARNING

Muscles are the parts of the body that get damaged most often, so they are most often in need of magnet therapy to speed recovery. But remember the warning from page 36: do not bring blood to a freshly torn muscle that is still bleeding internally.

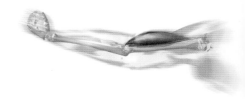

The push–pull mechanism of a muscle can be strained, sprained, or even torn.

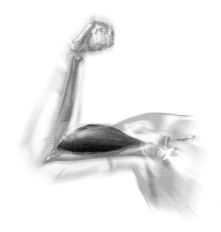

Magnets can be used to accelerate healing, but only after internal bleeding has stopped.

Using small adhesive magnets

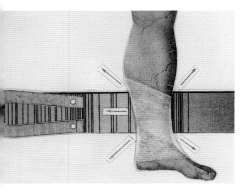

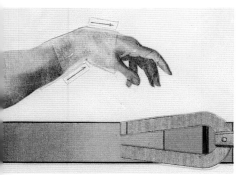

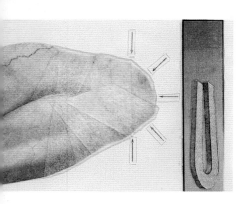

The placing of magnets depends on the injury and the individual. One on the site of the pain and a circle around it is usually effective.

We have looked at how magnets affect water and other fluids flowing through pipes. We have seen that the human body contains extensive pipework systems with fluids flowing through them. Because magnets can facilitate the flow of these liquids, they can have many beneficial effects on the body.

If the aim is to improve the flow of blood and the transportation of repair material to a site, use small adhesive magnets with the north—red or positive—pole against the skin. ("Small" in this case refers to the magnet's physical size; these magnets can range from 500 gauss to 8,000 gauss.) If the aim is to restrict flow, then place the south—blue or negative—pole of the magnet against the skin. Generally in magnetic therapy, a positive (red) side will stimulate, and a negative (blue) side will sedate or calm.

WHERE TO PUT THE MAGNETS

Choosing where to place magnets to improve fluid flows is not difficult. On large flattish areas, such as the abdomen or the thigh, find the center of the pain and place a magnet at that point; then find the outer edges of the painful area and place magnets around this edge, with about 1–1.5-inch (2–3-cm) gaps between the magnets. If the problem is a sprained wrist or ankle, then place the magnets in a band, again with gaps of about 1–1.5 inches (2–3 cm) around the affected limb about 3 inches (10 cm) above the damage. By above, I mean nearer the heart. If the wrist is damaged, the circle goes between wrist and elbow; if the elbow is painful, the arm should be encircled between elbow and shoulder. In cases of ankle injury, the circle goes between ankle and knee. For a knee injury, an evenly-spaced circle of magnets goes around the middle of the thigh.

As a general rule of thumb, leave the magnets in place for between 12 hours and 5 days (this, of course, depends on the injury). If the magnets get washed off in the bath or the shower, reapply them in the same position.

SPRAINS

In cases of sprained wrists, knees, or ankles, in addition to the band of magnets around a limb, try placing magnets on either side of the damaged part. Imagine a line or axis drawn through the joint, going through the center of the pain. The length of this line depends on the extent of the area of pain. Place your magnets at both the entry and exit points of this imaginary line. Use magnets that are around 600 gauss and remove them when relief has been obtained.

CRAMP

Cramp, pins and needles, and constant cold sensations are all indications of poor circulation. It is most advisable to consult a general practitioner to ensure that this poor circulation is not the result of some deterioration, restriction, or disease in the heart or vascular system.

Magnets can be used to relieve cramp and localized poor circulation. Encircle the limb about 8 inches (20 cm) above the place where the pain or discomfort is felt and leave the magnets in place for between two and five days. Again, by above, I mean the area between the discomfort and the heart.

Magnets have been found to be of particular benefit with cramp that occurs on one particular calf muscle at night. This painful condition often wakes the sufferer and disrupts sleep. The use of 800-gauss magnets in a circle around the thigh, about 2 inches (4 cm) above the knee with gaps of 1–1.5 inches (2–3 cm) between them, has brought great, and in some cases lasting, relief. They should be left in place until relief is obtained: this can be one night or as many as fourteen. If the cramp recurs and you have checked with your general practitioner that there is no serious overall problem, then reapply the magnets.

BROKEN BONES, IMPACT DAMAGE, OVERSTRETCHED MUSCLES

In cases of broken bones, impact damage, or overstretched muscles, similar applications will help. The object is to improve both the flow of repair material to the area and the removal of waste or damaged cells from the area. Magnets placed to improve blood and lymph flow will speed up recovery.

Magnets can be used between other physical treatment sessions, such as massage or shiatsu. Later in the book (see pages 90–91) I will go into detail about the use of magnets on acupuncture and pressure points, but it is worth remembering that between sessions, magnets can speed up the healing process.

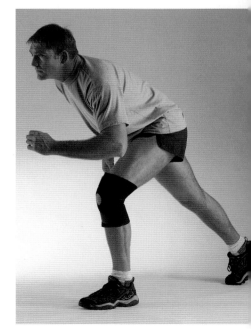

Supports with in-built magnetic strips have been used successfully both by amateur and professional sportspeople.

✳ | Using magnetized water

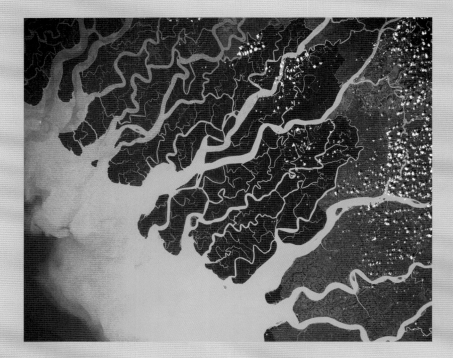

The delta of the River Ganges. There is an abundance of water on this planet, and much of it may be magnetized by the natural action of water flowing over rocks with magnetic properties.

Magnets applied to the exterior of pipes can improve water flows within the pipes. If the water itself can be affected by magnets, i.e. magnetized, before it enters the pipes, there may be further benefits. When water is magnetized, it does not mean that the water itself becomes magnetic, only that changes have taken place due to the influence of magnets.

HOW TO MAGNETIZE WATER

There are three ways to magnetize water. One is to trickle water slowly over a magnet on its way to a collection vessel. This mimics the natural effect of rivers, streams, or waterfalls seeping over lodestone or other naturally magnetic rocks. Another method is to place a magnet inside a jar of water and leave it for six to eight hours. The drawback to both these methods, however, is the risk of contamination of the water if any oxides or debris from the magnet enter the water, and therefore the person who consumes it.

A safer way is to stand a jar of water on a magnet and leave this for about 12 to 24 hours. Some magnet therapists advocate making up two jars, one that has the north pole touching the bottom of the jar, and the other that has the south pole in contact with the bottom of the jar. You can then mix some of the contents to form a third jar of bi-polar magnetized water. Quite large and powerful magnets are needed to magnetize water in this way—around 3,000 gauss—and the degree to which the water is affected by the magnets is almost impossible to quantify, unless you are doing this in a very specialized laboratory.

THE HEALING QUALITIES OF MAGNETIZED WATER

There are many claims made for the benefits of drinking magnetized water, but very little research has been done in the area. Reports in India suggest that magnetized water is beneficial for low blood pressure; it corrects any condition of imbalance. It also has a soothing, slightly sedative, effect on emotional upsets and is said to help normalize circulatory systems and improve energy levels. Some reports suggest it is helpful in the treatment of bronchial problems, including asthma and colds. The magnetized water should be taken in three daily doses, one before breakfast and the other two after meals. It is usual to use the bi-polar water, and each adult dose should be 2 fl oz (57 ml).

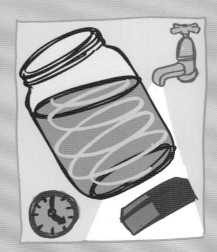

Magnetized water can also be used for washing wounds, eczema, sores, blemishes, etc. To relieve sore and tired eyes, try washing them in magnetized water, or soaking cotton-wool pads in the water. If you do drink any magnetized fluids or wash wounds in magnetized water, be sure that the very best hygiene practices have been observed and that the liquid you are using is free from all possible contamination.

Magnetized water has been credited with helping in the treatment of eating disorders, particularly anorexia. Indian reports suggest that two or three glasses of water a day removes the desire to suppress the appetite. Bi-polar water is also said to help relieve the pain of a headache and boost flagging energy levels.

Other liquids can also be magnetized and used in the same way as water. But because the body is 66 percent water, it seems logical that magnetized water will be best at improving liquid flows within the body.

One of the safest ways to make magnetized water in your own home is to stand a pitcher of water on a magnet. There are special beakers on the market too, which fulfill the same function.

✳ | Using large magnets

The therapeutic application of large magnets for relatively short periods of time (10 to 30 minutes) has a long history but is less common these days. Because of modern technical advances in magnet production, large magnets are being replaced with small and relatively powerful adhesive magnets and a range of magnetic support bandages. These smaller magnets can be held in position for longer periods than the large magnets.

HOW LARGE ARE LARGE MAGNETS?

Old-fashioned large magnets are thick disks about 4 in (10 cm) in diameter and 1.5–2 in (4–5 cm) thick. They have a capacity to "lift" 20 lbs (10 kg) of iron. Unfortunately there is no simple way of converting this information into a gauss or tesla figure, so this will not be attempted for the purposes of this book. With modern magnetic materials it is possible to make small magnets "lift" or "hold" 20 lbs (10 kg) of iron. The shape of the magnet and the materials it is made from rather than the actual gauss figure will influence the weight it can hold or lift. Some larger-sized magnets can have a very weak magnetic strength, while some small magnets can be quite powerful.

HOW TO USE LARGE MAGNETS

When large magnets are used, it is common to have two basic "styles": one for local treatment and the other for general treatment. For local treatment, place the magnet directly onto the troublesome spot, without any pressure. This can be taped on with medical tape, or plasters, or it can be held in place. If it is suspected that the problem has a bacterial cause, place the north-seeking pole against the skin, otherwise the south-seeking pole touches the skin. Some therapists prefer to place the north pole on one side of the problem area with the south pole opposite. Other therapists prefer to place one pole on the painful area and the opposite pole against the skin of the nearest extremity, i.e. the palm of a hand or the sole of a foot. For example, if the problem is in the right upper arm and involves swelling, then the north-seeking pole is placed over the problem area and the south-seeking pole is placed against the skin of the palm of the right hand. The magnets are left in place for 10 to 15 minutes—a shorter period for a child or very weak person.

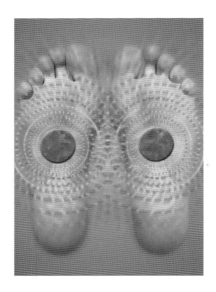

Large magnets can be placed on the soles of the feet to treat general discomfort, or an illness that is affecting the whole body.

LARGE MAGNETS FOR TREATING
GENERAL DISCOMFORT

To treat general discomfort, i.e. an illness not confined to one area of the body, place the magnets on the palms of the hands and the soles of the feet. If the illness is centered on the upper half of the body, place the magnets on the palms of the hands; if centered on the lower half, place the magnets on the soles of the feet. If the whole body is involved and in some way diseased, place magnets on the hands one day and on the feet the next day. The palms and soles are the end points of many branches of the general nervous system, so they are ideally suited for conducting the magnetic influence generated by the application of the magnets around the entire body via the nervous system network.

In some cases the north-seeking pole could be held against the front of the body while the south-seeking pole is placed on the back, physically opposite the other magnet. The therapist's decision as to the location of magnets on the body is determined by the unique aspects of each individual case.

The palms of the hands and the soles of the feet are the exit points for numerous branches of the nervous system, so are ideal points for general healing.

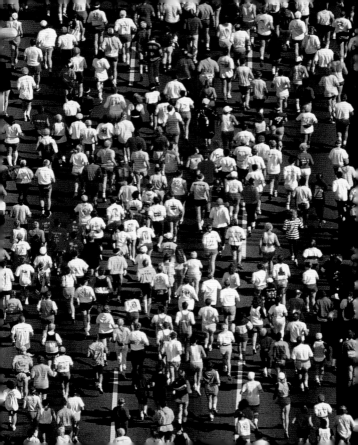

✳ | Chapter three

Specific healing We have already looked at the various ways in which magnetic influences can affect the body, from the surface of the skin down to cellular levels. In this section, we will explore more specific problems and find out how to use magnets and magnetic influences to help the body deal with these problems. But firstly we need to understand how the body deals with illness and disruption—its immune response.

The immune system is the body's main defense against attack from outside organisms such as bacteria and viruses. The publicity surrounding AIDS and HIV has brought the immune system into public focus, but it is remarkable how few people realize that many other illnesses are the result of a degenerating or malfunctioning immune system that actually attacks the body. We will examine, very briefly, the human immune system and see how we can help our bodies in the fight to prevent or overcome ill-health.

We will also look at ways to use magnets to speed up recovery from broken bones, sports injuries, sprains, and circulation problems. There are specific case examples of how magnets have helped overcome the pain of such afflictions as night cramps, stiff shoulders, and inflexible knees.

The immune system

The HIV virus that causes AIDS, as it looks under a microscope.

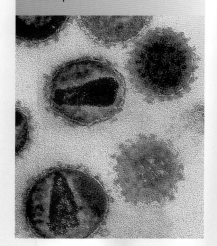

The body's defense system is made up of various arrangements of cells and molecules that work together to destroy invading organisms. The invading molecules come from various sources, usually bacterium, and are called antigens— the antigens are any substance that the body regards as "foreign" or potentially dangerous. Antibodies are produced by the body in response to this attack: these are a special type of blood protein that is synthesized in the lymphoid tissue. They circulate in the plasma to attack the antigen and render it harmless. In addition to these, the immune system also has specialized cells called antigen-presenting cells, which, at a cellular level, actually contain the substances that the body considers to be a threat. This "contamination" of these cells allows them to ingest antigens and fragment them. The most common types of antigen-presenting cells are macrophages. These are the healing and repairing agents. Once an antigen has been ingested and broken up, fragments, called antigenic peptides, are released. These join up with molecules known as major histocompatibility complex (MHC), which are specialized to stick to the outside of these invading molecules and help identify them to the defense system. This alerts the whole defensive system to the fact that an invader has been engaged and enables it to recognize that invader. Some white blood cells, known as T lymphocytes, are specialists in the recognition of invaders, and as various models of T lymphocytes can recognize different types of invaders, they set off signals that start the rest of the immune system going.

Antibiotics were developed to kill the kind of bacteria that have been described above. However, overuse of antibiotics can lead to a situation where the bacteria present are not fully killed off and new strains have evolved that can resist the chemicals originally used to eradicate them.

THE LYMPHATIC SYSTEM

Infectious agents can get into the body at any point, so our defense system has well-connected lookouts posted around the whole body, a bit like fortresses or castles linked together by defended roads. This defensive lookout network is called the lymphatic system and it can spring into action when required to fend off an invasion. Bones, the spleen, the thymus, blood, and skin all play some part in the defense structure, but the lymphatic—or lymph—system has the major role.

Lymphocytes, a type of white blood cell with responsibility for specific immunity, are made in the primary lymphoid organs. The thymus, a lymphoid organ near the base of the neck, makes T lymphocyte cells; bone marrow, a tissue that is the source of most blood cells, produces B lymphocytes. Lymphocytes flow around in the blood stream until they settle down in other lymph nodes (often called glands). They reside there until they are called upon to rush out of the nodes to deal with invaders. Many parts of this lymphoid system also have other work to do as well as fighting infection. For example, the thyroid gland produces hormones that regulate the growth and development of the body. Problems occur when this complex system goes wrong. For instance, when the thyroid gland becomes overactive and sends too much of a particular hormone into the bloodstream, various organs take up these hormonal messengers and cause undesirable bodily responses, such as sweating, overeating, bad temper, and tiredness. Underactivity of the thyroid also causes problems, such as tiredness, aches and pains, forgetfulness, sensitivity to cold, and weight gain.

HOW WE CAN HELP

To enable our body to be constantly vigilant to the invasion of harmful organisms, we can do several things: we can provide the chemical ingredients the defenses need by eating fresh foods that contain the correct balance of protein, vitamins, and minerals; we can ensure that the transportation infrastructure of the body is working well by getting regular exercise; and we can avoid situations that overload and therefore weaken the immune system, such as excessive intake of alcohol or drugs, excessive mental stress, or excessive physical activity.

HOW MAGNETS HELP THE IMMUNE SYSTEM

Magnets can be used to stimulate blood flow and thereby improve the transmission of healing and repairing agents. They can be used to speed up the assimilation of beneficial chemicals by the blood by improving the flow of digestive secretions. (Use small 600–800 gauss magnets on acupuncture points St36, Sp6, and LI4.) (*For all acupuncture points mentioned throughout the book, please refer to pages 108–121 for detailed diagrams and information.*)

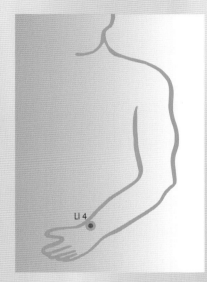

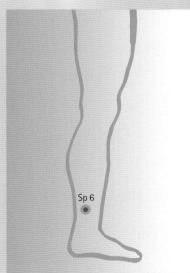

These points can be used to improve the flow of the digestive secretions, which in turn affect the whole body.

Fractures and broken bones

BROKEN LIMBS

A broken leg has several unwanted side effects aside from the pain and inconvenience. Because the damaged part must not be subjected to loads or weights, the muscles around it are used less. This leads, very quickly, to muscle wastage and loss of fitness, strength, and mobility. The longer the injury takes to heal, the worse things get. Another side effect is a shift in posture. Some people who have a broken leg change their posture so much that they can distort the hip joint and throw their pelvic girdle out of alignment. If this change in posture is extreme and is held for too long, there can be damage to the lower abdominal organs.

There are several types of broken bones, from a simple fracture in the center of a long bone, with the two ends still in line and barely separated, to the multiple fracture, with dislocation at a junction with a multiple action joint. In all cases, it is important to get the parts in the correct position relative to each other. Usually this is achieved by physical manipulation followed by enforced movement restriction. Applying a plaster cast or binding the limb to some rigid apparatus is usually sufficient in most cases. In more complex fractures, it is necessary to use internally positioned rods, screws, or wires. In all these cases, the objective is the same: to hold the parts together until a natural mending of the broken bone takes place. The healing process involves some slight change to the exterior surface of the bone, possibly with some slight swellings around the line of the fracture.

The repair process requires blood. Blood brings the nutrients such as vitamin C, which is essential for repair work, to the site and takes away unwanted waste particles. The flow of blood is what enables the natural mending process to take place. Once it has been established that an increased flow of blood will be beneficial and not damaging—as it would be if the blood vessels were also fractured and there was internal or external bleeding—magnets can be used to speed up the flow of blood to and from the damage site. This, in turn, will help to speed up the recovery process.

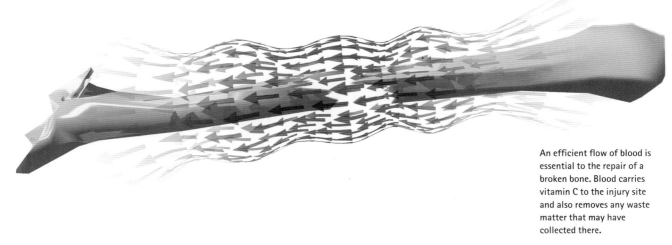

An efficient flow of blood is essential to the repair of a broken bone. Blood carries vitamin C to the injury site and also removes any waste matter that may have collected there.

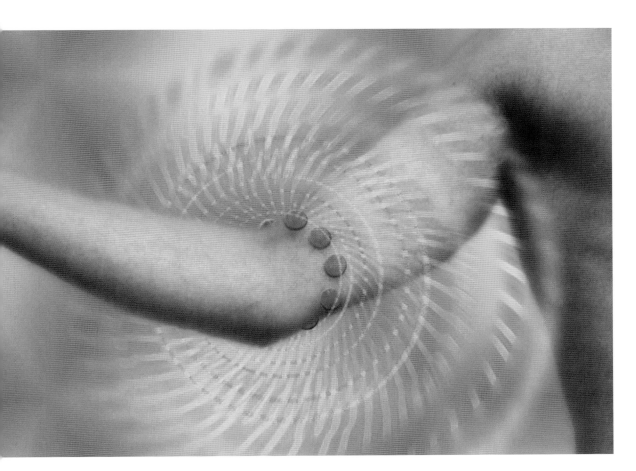

As long as there is no bleeding and the bones are correctly positioned, magnets can be placed at 1-inch (2-cm) intervals in a circle around the afflicted limb, between the fracture and the heart. If possible, also place a magnet on the surface of the skin over the site of a fracture. However, the thickness of a plaster will prevent a magnet placed over the site from having much effect, so for plastered joints, this method will be ineffective. But in situations where plaster has not been applied, such as a cracked bone, magnets can be applied directly over the site. Some people believe that magnets placed as close as possible to a fracture site, particularly if encircling it, will improve the strength of the actual rejoining.

Encircling the broken or fractured limb with magnets can help the healing process, as long as it is unplastered. The magnets should be positioned as close to the break as possible.

✳ | Sports injuries

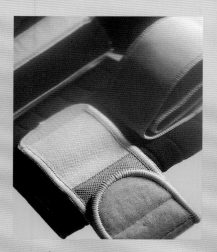

Magnetic wraps and supports are available for all joints, as well as for larger areas such as the back, head, and shoulders.

MAGNETIC WRAPS

Most sports participants will need, at some time or another, to apply an external support to a trouble site. This may be the site of a previous injury or a place where there always seems to be weakness, or pain, or both. Usually some sort of bandage is wrapped around the injury. The supporting wrap needs to allow flexibility, while protecting and supporting where this is needed.

Modern magnet therapy wraps have magnets or magnetic strips bonded into fabric and are wrapped around and fastened with Velcro. The wraps are designed to suit particular joints or areas of the body; a wrist support will not go around the thigh, and a thigh support would be too bulky to use on a wrist. They also come in various sizes to suit the wearer.

THE PHASES OF TREATMENT

There are several phases in the treatment of a sports injury: immediate first aid, if the injury is instantly evident; pain reduction and mobility enhancement; recovery; and finally rehabilitation followed by full recovery. All of this can take much longer than anticipated; however, by applying magnets to the injury, total recovery time can be decreased. Place one 600–800 gauss magnet at the center of the painful area and then encircle the area with small magnets placed 1 in (2–3 cm) apart. The magnets will increase blood-flow rates and the lymphatic circulation.

TENNIS ELBOW

Injuries to the points where muscles are joined to the skeleton are most common. Tennis elbow is a common injury among all sports enthusiasts who use their arms. Hitting a tennis ball traveling at 30 miles (50 km) per hour is theoretically equivalent to lifting a weight of 55 lbs (25 kg). If the forces are not distributed evenly throughout the body but are concentrated at one point—for example, at the junction of the muscle to the bone, at the outer side of the elbow—the result is tennis elbow. It is estimated that 45 percent of tennis players who play every day and 25 percent of those who play twice a week suffer from tennis elbow. It is more common when the players are over 40 years old. This injury can be prevented by using playing techniques that distribute the load evenly.

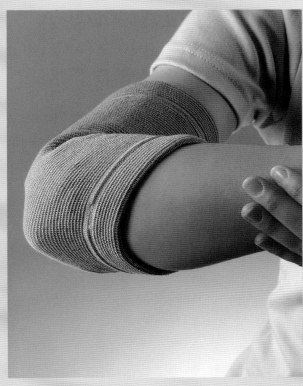

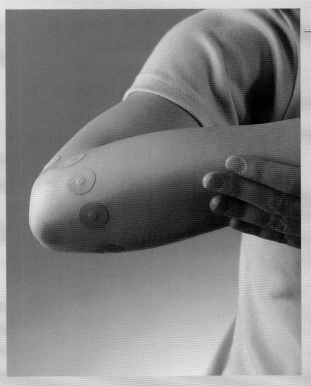

A special tennis elbow
support, containing magnets,
can be purchased to help
ease an injury.

Alternatively, the elbow
injury can be encircled with
600–800 gauss magnets to
obtain relief from the pain.

There is not normally swelling in cases of tennis elbow, so if swelling is present it is vital to get a full medical diagnosis before you begin to think about using magnet therapy. To reduce the pain, cool the injury for two days and then apply alternating hot and cold compresses. Apply specific elbow magnetic support bandages and rest the damaged area. You can continue with other activitites, including tennis, as long as you avoid the action that aggravates the injury.

BURSITIS

Bursitis is the inflammation of a bursa—a sac or pouchlike cavity that usually contains fluid that reduces friction between a tendon and a bone. Bursitis is usually the result of some form of impact—a fall or blow—and involves swelling and bleeding. The bleeding is often internal, so the use of heat and/or magnets should be avoided for several days, until there is no danger of fresh bleeding. This may take up to seven days. After initial first aid and rest for seven to ten days, a magnetic support bandage may be beneficial.

✳ | Pain

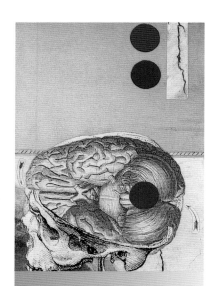

The way that the brain perceives pain differs greatly from person to person. Do not ignore it, however unimportant it appears.

THE PAIN OF HEALING

Pain due to the healing process, i.e. pain that is felt while healing is taking place, can be difficult to overcome. When faced with such things as postoperative pain, it is not wise to use anything that will bring more blood to the wound site until all risk of bleeding from severed or ruptured blood vessels has passed. Once the vessels have been sealed, magnets may be placed on the site to help reduce any pain and swelling that may be present.

The dictionary describes pain as the sensation of acute physical hurt or discomfort caused by injury, illness, etc. Quantifying the pain an individual feels is a very difficult problem. We all have different levels at which we experience discomfort and hurt as "painful"—the so-called pain threshold. People with high pain thresholds should not dismiss others as weaklings. The level of pain felt by each individual is real, and the reactions to that pain are valid for that person.

Different parts of our body have different numbers of nerve receptors that relay pain messages to the brain; so the same discomfort at two different areas of the body may result in a greater sensation of pain at one place than at the other.

The level of injury and discomfort that one person finds unbearable could be acceptable to another. Our mental attitudes and emotional conditioning influence these levels of acceptability. Childbirth is an extremely painful process and yet women voluntarily repeat it. It is accepted that this is a normal part of life and that this great but relatively short-term pain will end with the joy of birth. This knowledge helps to make this level of pain acceptable.

The amount of emotion-linked hormones and other chemicals rushing about in our bodies also affect how we experience pain. Adrenaline is so busy making us active that it can override the pain receptors, temporarily. The body can produce its own version of morphine, which can dull or temporarily delay the sensations of pain. This also differs from individual to individual.

Pain may be caused by a long-term illness or by a physical injury. Individuals who participate in high-risk sports, such as skiing, may become more used to severe pain than other people.

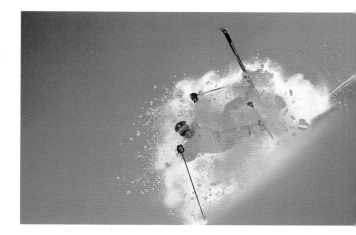

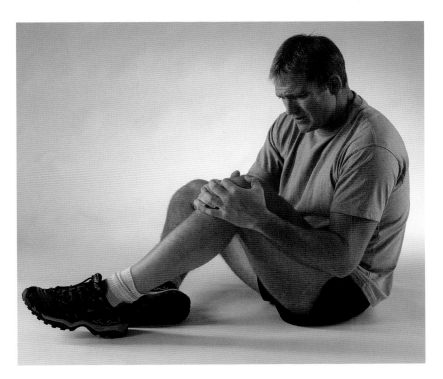

It may be tempting to mask the pain of a sports-related injury with painkillers. This is ultimately self-defeating, and may cause problems.

PAIN AS A MESSENGER

When any part of the body is subjected to something that is actually or potentially damaging, signals are sent to the brain. The brain registers this as pain. The purpose of this reaction is to stop the body from continuing on the course of action that is causing the damage. Pain is part of the natural defense mechanisms; pain is telling you something is being damaged. It may be that the "damage" is actually repair work to previously disorganized tissue; it may be that lazy muscles are being asked to relearn activities and they regard this activity as "damage." But in all cases, the body is telling you something, and you should heed the message.

Magnets can help to alleviate pain by improving the flow of nutrients to the injury and speeding up the repair of damaged tissue. They can also reduce the pressure that is applied to nerve endings in cases of swelling that are not due to internal bleeding. Magnets can also be used to relieve headaches and migraine.

✳ | Chronic pain

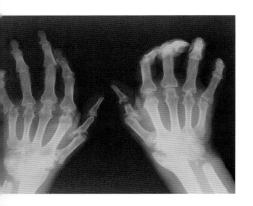

Rheumatoid arthritis is a crippling and debilitating disease. The swelling and pain associated with it may be eased by magnet therapy.

Chronic, or long-term pain, is very damaging. The prospect of constant pain and its restrictions on normal life and activities has a very detrimental physical and emotional effect. Chronic pain is often due to the deterioration of the bones or tissues of the body. Magnets can help by stimulating the flow of repair materials to the damaged area. However, this assumes that the blood contains these repair materials, which are acquired through a healthy diet and good digestion, and that the blood is a good-quality transporter itself.

TREATING CHRONIC PAIN WITH MAGNETS

For chronic pain, apply magnets to the local site of the pain, one in the center and others encircling the area. These should be left on for ten days, then removed for a week: repeat this process until the pain eases. The effect could be enhanced by the use of magnets on suitable acupuncture points: LI4, Sp6, and St36 are the usual ones for chronic pain although this will have to be adjusted to the individual. The most usual strength magnets for this purpose are 600 gauss. However, the strength of the magnets used depends on the nature, depth, and severity of the pain and will differ from person to person. If in doubt, consult your therapist.

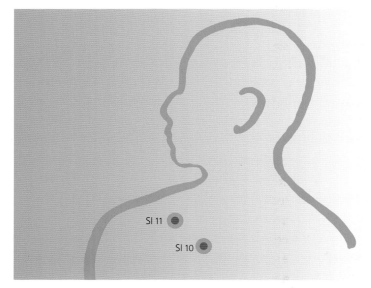

SI 11

SI 10

Localized pain and stiffness in the arms and shoulders can be eased by stimulating Small Intestine points 10 and 11.

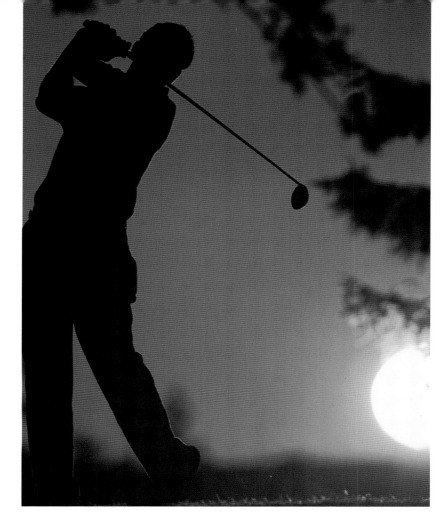

Many golfers, both amateur and professional, use magnet therapy to help with repetitive strain injury.

TREATING ARTHRITIS AND RHEUMATISM

The chronic nature of arthritic and rheumatoid pain can be very debilitating. Arthritis is a degeneration of the cartilage and/or a disturbance to the synovial membranes (these normally prevent two bones from being in direct and painful contact with each other). The result is usually swelling and pain. Analgesics are commonly used to combat the swelling and reduce the pain. Magnets placed in circles around the affected joint, one circle above and one below, can help in the same way. Magnets of 600 gauss strength can be used but this will vary from patient to the patient. Try keeping the magnets on for ten days and then removing them for a week. This routine will need to be repeated until relief is obtained. Again, if in doubt, consult your therapist.

Rheumatoid pain affects joints, muscles, or fibrous tissue and has many causes. Massage and magnets can help improve blood flow through muscles and remove the crystalline debris that is a common cause of rheumatoid pain. Eating oily fish or taking fish-oil supplements will help in the longer term. Place one magnet in the center of the local site of pain and a circle of magnets around the area. Magnets of 600–800 gauss strength can be used as before.

Circulation problems

Garlic and oily fish, both beneficial foods, can help circulation problems, and are also beneficial to general well-being in the long term.

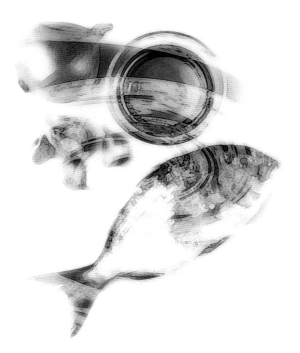

Cramp, that odd sensation generally known as "pins and needles," coldness in fingers and toes, and numbness in localized areas are all symptoms of poor circulation. When circulation is poor, energy levels are low and the muscles are weak and painful, especially when participating in exercise and sports.

Poor circulation is often caused by stress, but it may also be an inherited problem. In cases of poor circulation, it is especially important that the blood's ability to carry oxygen and nutrients is at its maximum. Exercise will improve the blood's oxygen-carrying abilities, but avoid sudden movement when cold or when muscles are strained in any way. Yoga helps to free up tense and restricted joints and muscles, thereby freeing up circulation. A healthy diet is needed to supply all the required nutrients. Generous amounts of root ginger and garlic in the diet will also be beneficial in the long term. Magnets, by improving blood flow, will reduce the effects of poor circulation and ease localized discomfort. Encircle the troublesome spot, placing the magnets between it and the heart. Use magnets of 600–800 gauss and leave them in place for seven to ten days, or until circulation has improved. In chronic cases, try leaving the magnets on for ten days then removing them for a week—repeat this routine until relief is obtained.

POSSIBLE CAUSES

A medical checkup to ensure that poor circulation is not due to a problem with the heart or blood vessels is the first step. This is very important in all cases, but particularly when there is a sudden numbness in a localized area.

CASE STUDY 1

A lively woman of 75 revealed that her sleep was often disturbed by cramp pains in the left calf muscle. A circle of 800-gauss magnets, roughly 2 inches (4 cm) apart, was attached to the leg about 4 inches (10 cm) above the left knee with the north-seeking pole against the skin. They were held in place with adhesive medical tape and every effort was made to ensure that the tape did not in any way restrict either blood flow or muscular movement. The magnets were left in place for five days and nights; if washed off they were replaced, maintaining the same position. After this time, the woman reported that she was no longer being woken by the pain at night; she was enjoying a full night's sleep. The magnets were removed and she has found that the condition has not returned.

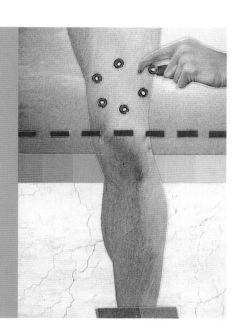

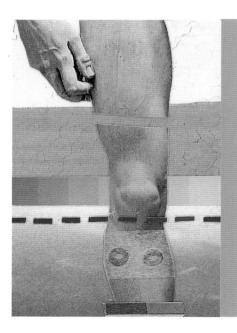

CASE STUDY 2

A 35-year-old man who works at a computer for long hours complained that he suffered from cramp during exercise. He enjoyed playing football and saw it as a way of giving his body much-needed exercise. After about 30 minutes of sporadic running, he would get painful twinges in the left calf muscle. Magnets (600–800 gauss) were taped around the leg just about 1 inch (2–3 cm) below the fold of the knee. They were placed in position about an hour before exercise was due to start and removed after the exercise. Because sweat tended to remove the tape, it was replaced with a support bandage that held the magnets in place. While the patient did not become fit overnight, he was able to play without the pain.

✳ | Migraine, headaches, and asthma

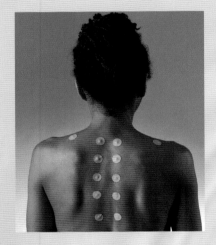

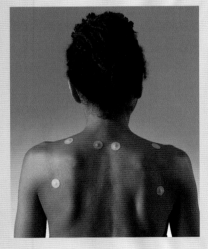

Small magnets can be attached to specific acupuncture points near the spine to relieve the distressing symptoms of asthma (top). Migraines can be treated with magnets applied to the acupuncture points depicted above.

MIGRAINES

There are various different types of migraine. In classic migraine, the attack is usually preceded by an "aura," a sensation that may be different for each sufferer. Other preceding symptoms may include numbness or weakness on one side of the body; bright, white, or colored shapes, spots, or lines before the eyes; or problems such as double vision and blind spots in the vision. These signs may last for up to half an hour before the attack begins. When there is no aura, the condition is termed common migraine. Symptoms, however, do vary from person to person.

As every person is different, so there is no standardized magnet therapy for migraines; however, the application of 600 to 800 gauss magnets is effective in many cases. The following collection of acupuncture points help to restore balance to the energy system. Attach a row of magnets 1 in (2.5 cm) apart along both sides of the spine, between the spine and the shoulder blade. The top magnet should be level with the top of the shoulder blade, and the bottom one roughly in line with the bottom of the shoulder blade.

Magnets can also be placed on the legs at acupuncture point St36, on the hands at LI4, on the head, on both sides, in line with the outer extremity of the eye halfway between the corner of the eye and the ear; also over the top of the eyebrow in the middle of each eyebrow. In many cases, magnets on L3 and GB43 have also been helpful in the restoration of balance and energy to the system. The position of magnets will depend on the individual and the type of migraine symptoms you are experiencing. Consult your therapist for more information.

HEADACHES

Headaches can be very severe, but unlike migraines there is no nausea or sight distortion. Headaches can be caused by the same things that cause migraines, or they can be caused by impact—trauma—damage to the head. (Migraines that are triggered by impact would be very rare but this might occur if there was a latent propensity toward migraine-suffering in the victim. The shock that is caused by or that accompanies any physical impact could also trigger a migraine.) To treat headaches, place magnets on the acupuncture points as for migraine, but the St36 point can be omitted as headaches are not normally accompanied by an imbalance in the digestive energy. Use a magnetic headband wrapped—but not too tightly—around the forehead to replace the head-positioned magnets described for migraine. (A migraine sufferer would need to be more precise in the placement of magnets so a headband would be less useful.) If the headache is localized, the following points are recommended: the lower part of the back of the head, the occipital region; GB20, UB60, and SI3 both sides: front of the head; St8, LI4, St44 both sides: one side of the head (treat the side that hurts); GB8, TW5, GB41.

Use magnets of 600–800 gauss and leave them in place until the pain passes. This might take up to five days but most people do not allow a headache to incapacitate them and probably would not go about their everyday lives with visible magnets in place.

ASTHMA

The incidence of asthma does seem to be increasing, but some caution is required when examining the statistics. Many cases that twenty years ago would not have been recorded are now being diagnosed as asthma. An explanation for this change may be the fact that asthma is now seen as a treatable illness, so it is acceptable to label a set of symptoms as asthma. But this does not fully explain the increases. Countries such as Australia and New Zealand with relatively unpolluted environments have recorded increasing levels of asthma. International figures suggests that it is a disease of the developed world. Some people have pointed to house mites, pets, smoking, and a more toxic environment to explain the increased levels. But no research can fully explain why asthma has become more prevalent.

Asthma attacks are triggered by a variety of situations: stress, cold winds, changes in diet, hot dry climatic conditions, and high pollen counts. The application of magnets to the following acupuncture points may help reduce the severity of the attack: UB13, LU7, LU5, LU1, LI4, CV22, and St 40. Use 600 to 800 gauss magnets and leave them in place for at least three days. Once an attack has started, apply magnets to UB20 and UB43, as well as the above-mentioned points. If the lung function is generally weak, magnets on UB13, LU9, and St36 may help. These points are used to rebalance the energy within the patient; generally, prevention is much easier than the actual treatment of a symptomatic condition.

ASTHMA ATTACKS

Magnets can help relieve the symptoms of asthma and prevent severe attacks; however, it is vital that asthma sufferers should continue taking their prescribed medications even when using magnet therapy techniques.

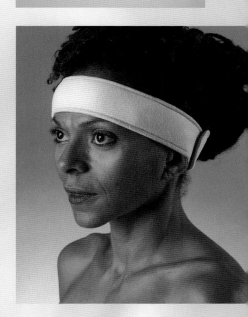

A magnetic headband can be worn to provide relief from mild to severe headaches.

✳ | Insomnia

The most common cause of insomnia is stress, and in particular stress that is caused by emotional disturbance. Even once the disturbance has been alleviated or removed, the symptoms of insomnia may continue to persist. Insomnia can also be a conditioned reaction. This is particularly the case for those who suffer from bad nightmares or those who expect to be woken during the night and train their bodies and minds to avoid too deep a sleep. Parents with new babies may recognize this problem! Also, if you are bored with your life and feel that there is nothing to wake up for, this can also cause insomnia. It may sound paradoxical but if we do not have an incentive to wake up and get going, then there is no incentive to sleep soundly. If you do often wake up in the night and cannot get back to sleep, then it is best to get out of bed and not lie there worrying about not being able to sleep. Train yourself to realize that your bed is a place of rest and avoid drinking tea or coffee after 6 p.m. if you are prone to insomnia.

On the other hand, sleeping for too long has been found to be counterproductive too. The metabolic rate can slow down and induce a feeling of tired sluggishness. It is better to get up after eight hours sleep and maybe have a nap later in the day than to sleep solidly for ten to twelve hours at a stretch.

USING MAGNETS TO IMPROVE SLEEP

Magnets can help promote a more relaxing and therefore more beneficial sleep. This may not necessarily mean a longer sleep but a deeper, less restless, period of slumber that will ensure we wake up refreshed and ready to face the day. Specialized mattresses and mattress covers (overlays) that have magnetized strips built into them can be very beneficial. Suppliers of these items have had many glowing reports from satisfied customers. Pillows with magnets built into them are also available. Most of these pieces of equipment use 800 gauss magnets. Small adhesive magnets placed on the acupuncture points UB15, UB19, UB23, K3, GB12, and St36 will also help. Put the magnets in place about an hour before going to bed and keep them on during the night.

Pain can also disrupt sleep, and night cramps are a common problem. Check up on the sections of this book that discuss these problems (pages 62–67) and use magnets as suggested to remove these potential causes of a sleepless night.

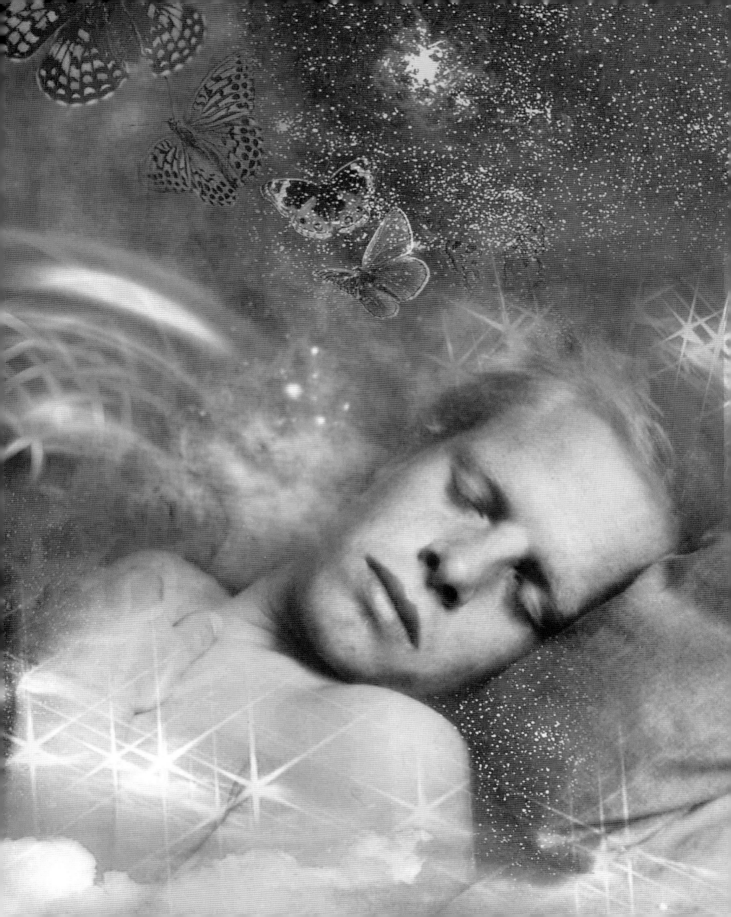

✳ | Anxiety

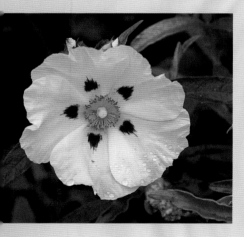

Flower remedies, and in particular Rescue Remedy, can be used in tandem with magnet therapy to help anxiety and stress. Rock Rose is one of the constituents of Rescue Remedy.

Anxiety is a very distressing condition. It can be triggered by straightforward, known physical causes, such as vertigo (standing on a mountain top and being afraid of falling), claustrophobia (fear of being in a small space), or indeed living with a violent or unpredictable person. These types of anxiety have direct, known causes and can only be eased by either avoiding the situation that causes the discomfort, or seeking specialized treatment for phobias. Anxiety with less obvious causes, such as emotional trauma or torment, is an altogether different thing to deal with. This can be a bottomless pit of blame, self-doubt, and guilt into which it is possible to disappear when everything seems to fail and we think that everything is our fault. A ladder is needed to climb out of this pit but experience has shown that the sufferer's family—who should be best placed to provide that ladder—are sadly often a part of the problem.

What is needed is a way to show the sufferer that he or she is a worthwhile person, who can face the future, who is competent, and therefore can cope with anxiety. Everyone suffers from some kind of fear and anxiety. These are normal and natural feelings, but problems arise when a person becomes so trodden down by them as to be unable to function properly and so not able to overcome the feelings. It is important to work hard to show the person that he or she is worthwhile. It is also important to empower sufferers so they are able to recover themselves, and this can in turn relieve listlessness and lack of energy. Although the role of close relatives and loved ones is crucial—and this cannot be stressed enough—it is often the case that they seem to wish to keep the sufferer subservient, or at least appear to resist any attempt at empowerment. People with anxiety are often on the receiving end of someone else's attempts to control a situation. The person in question must be allowed to develop self-esteem and a sense of self-worth, which will enable him or her to deal with the anxiety themselves.

The symptoms of anxiety can be very wide-ranging and include sweating, palpitations, difficulty in breathing, sleeplessness, irritability, loss of appetite, overeating, overindulgence generally, loss of willpower, loss of concentration, and all the usual manifestations of fear. Hyperventilation and convulsions are also possible symptoms and can be dangerous for the victim and very worrying for family members. Seek immediate medical help if this occurs.

If you suffer from anxiety, it is important to relax and take time out for yourself. Yoga, massage, shiatsu, and aromatherapy can all relieve suffering and may enable the victim to identify the cause of the anxiety and then deal with it.

The use of 600 to 800 gauss magnets on the following acupuncture points can help severe physical symptoms that are caused by anxiety: UB12, UB20, UB21, CV6, CV14, H7, P6, St40, and GB34. Try to leave the magnets in place for between seven to ten days, and reapply them if they get washed off.

Flower remedies can also help: Aspen, Banana, Cherry Plum, Filagree, Mimulus, Rock Rose, and Strawberry Cactus can ease varying feelings of anxiety. However, a combination of remedies can be a great help. Conscious care of yourself or the anxious person in question can provide a definite boost for self-esteem.

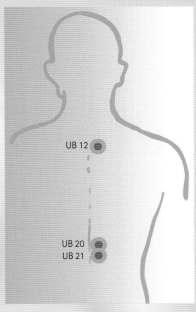

UB 12

UB 20
UB 21

Physical symptoms of anxiety—palpitations, breathlessness, and irritability—can be eased by stimulating these acupuncture points.

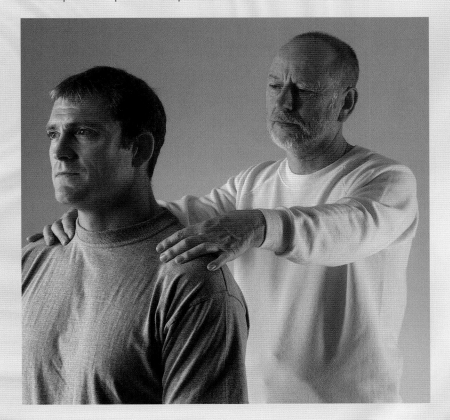

A full shiatsu massage is relaxing in itself, and may help an individual address their fear and discover the root of their anxiety.

Lower back pain, morning sickness, and the common cold

LOWER BACK PAIN

LOWER BACK PAIN

Medical examination, particularly of the kidneys and kidney functions, is advisable in all cases of lower back pain. Manipulative correction may be required if the bone structure or muscular anchorages have been disturbed in some way.

Magnetic bandages and supports are widely available and very useful in the treatment of lower back pain. Spot magnets of 600–800 gauss can be applied to the local area of the pain: one magnet in the center and the others encircling it. The size of this circle depends on the size of the patient and the extent of the painful area. The use of magnets on the following points may also help: GV3, GV4, K3, UB23, UB52, UB58.

For lower back pain, the center of the pain may be encircled by small magnets, or acupuncture points (as here) can be stimulated instead.

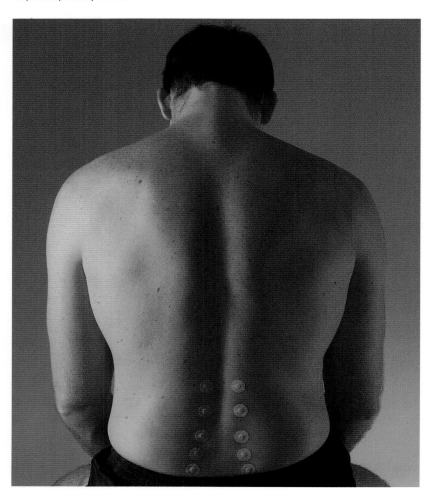

MORNING SICKNESS

It is considered unwise to use magnets, especially strong magnets, near the developing baby. The effects are unknown, so it is wise to be extra cautious. The specific acupuncture point Sp6 should also be avoided. While there is no evidence that the normally available magnets are of sufficient strength to do harm, it is best to be cautious. Use small magnets (600 to 800 gauss maximum) on points P6 and St36 only to relieve the symptoms of morning sickness.

In morning sickness, the pressure of the magnet on the point is possibly as much a part of the remedy as the magnet itself: keep it on or remove it and reapply it as required. Each individual reacts differently to the hormonal changes and imbalances that result in morning sickness, so it is not possible to be precisely prescriptive about treatment.

COMMON COLD

Magnets will not kill off viruses but they can help improve our resilience and therefore our recovery time; they can also help relieve symptoms and help us cope while the body fights off the invading virus.

When suffering from the "heavy head," apply magnets to the acupuncture points suggested for headaches. For general relief of cold symptoms, apply small (600 to 1,000 gauss) magnets to the following points for four to five days: Lu1, Lu7, CV16, UB12, UB20, LI4, K7, and on any particularly sore local point.

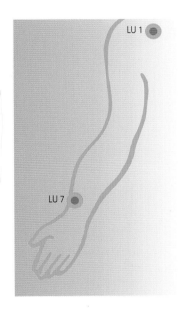

For a cold, magnets can be used on any tender spots and on Lu1 and Lu7, among other acupuncture points, to relieve the general symptoms.

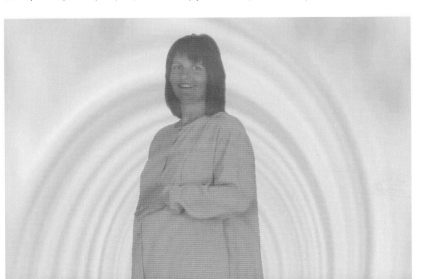

Magnets can be used during pregnancy, but they must be kept away from the developing baby. Sp6 must be particularly avoided.

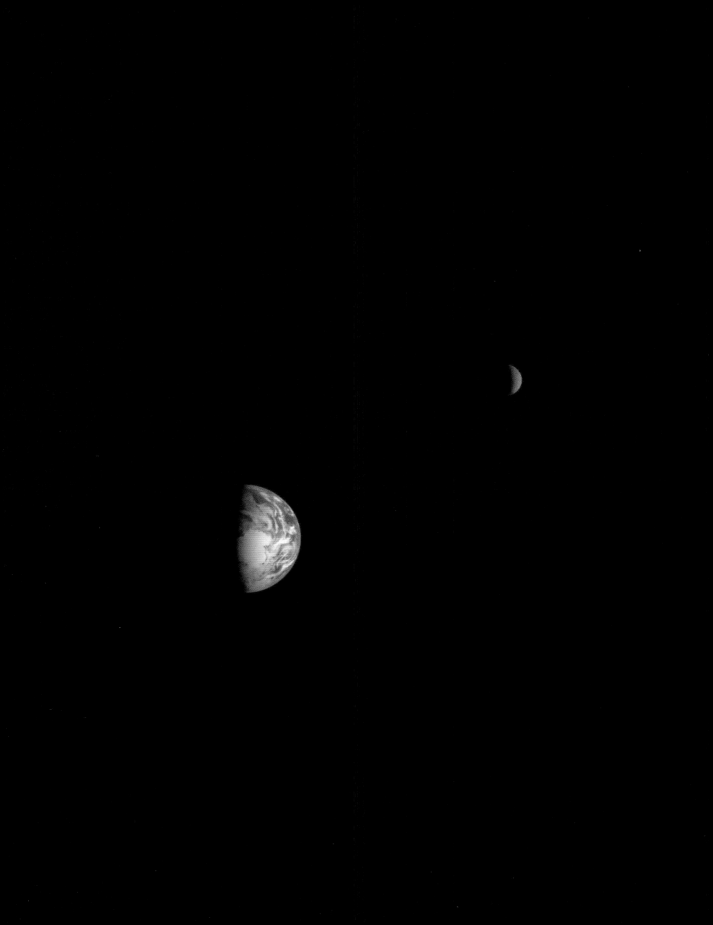

✳ | Chapter four

Magnetic influences We have already seen how magnetism and magnets can be used for healing and pain control. In this chapter, we will look at other aspects of magnetism—its connection with and influence on myths, ley lines, and dreams. We will also examine how magnets can be used to enhance other forms of treatment, such as flower remedies, homeopathy, shiatsu, and acupuncture. Finally, we will discuss simple magnetic experiments that you can try at home.

✳ | Magnets and myths

Our ancestors could sense, but not fully understand, the forces of magnetism that rule the universe by governing the relations between the stars, the earth, and all the planets. This mysterious force, and the wonder it inspired, may be at the root of many ancient myths that are still told today.

MERLIN AND MAGNETISM

The Celtic mythical figure of Merlin (Myrddin) is often depicted carrying a magic staff or sword. According to legend, Merlin locked the sword Excalibur into a rock, so that only the chosen one could remove it. Did Merlin know the secrets of magnetism? Was he able to lock Excalibur into a magnetic hold? When Arthur, his protégé, was ready to take on a leadership role, Merlin could have somehow brought a "like" pole to the rock so that the sword was repelled when Arthur pulled it. This magical event may have a magnetic explanation.

Merlin is said in some myths to have taken the 13 treasures of Britain with him when he sailed away. Among these was a sword called Dyrnwyn, which had

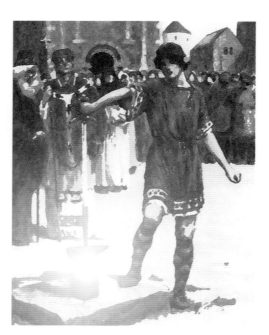

magical powers only Merlin could use safely. Another treasure was Cadair, a chair that would take those who sat on it anywhere they wished to go. Tawlbwrdd was a board game in which the pieces moved themselves and Modrwy was a ring that conferred invisibility on the wearer. Merlin is said to have carried a staff that could deflect arrows. All of these wondrous powers could be explained in terms of magnetism, and its powers of attraction and repulsion.

Was Merlin a master of magnetism? Many of his magical powers can be explained in terms of magnets and their properties.

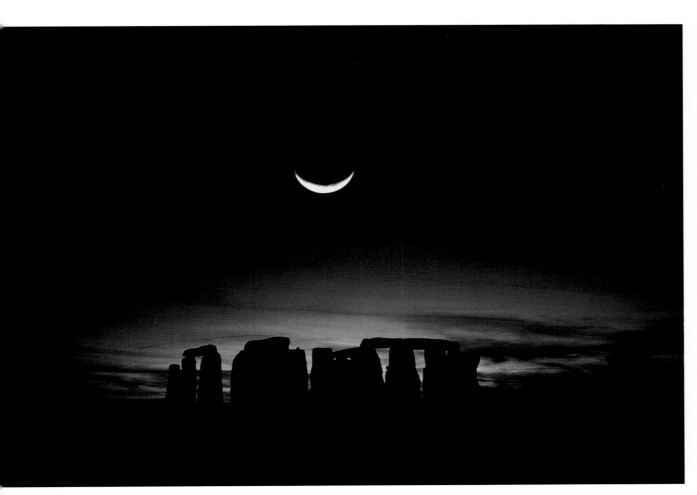

STONEHENGE

Merlin is said by some to have been the engineer responsible for Stonehenge. To this day, it remains a puzzle how such huge stones could have been transported to the site and erected using the technology available at the time. Perhaps Merlin knew how to use magnetic forces to transport the stones along ley lines. But in order to maintain his status as a great wizard, he may have kept his knowledge to himself and cloaked his abilities in an aura of magic.

The monoliths that make up the enigma that is Stonehenge, England, may have been transported to their resting places along ley lines.

✳ | Ley lines

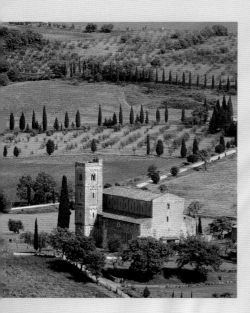

It has been suggested that churches were often built at the junction of ley lines.

The old English word *ley* means "arable land temporarily under grass." The age-old method of crop rotation meant that for one growing season a plot of land was left fallow, or unused, so it could recover. Grass would grow and be used as animal food the following year. "Ley" referred to land that was naturally recovering. The dictionary definition of a ley line is a line joining two prominent points in a landscape, thought to coincide with a prehistoric track. This raises the question of how, in a period when much of the country was uncultivated and covered with forest, did people navigate and create these tracks? Wouldn't it have been simpler to follow streams and rivers?

The answer may lie in the combination of the word "ley" and ancient navigation methods. If our ancient forebears could somehow sense natural lines of magnetic influence, and they associated these with the land that was peaceful and in recovery, then the term "ley lines" becomes significant. To follow some intuitively understood pathway that was secure and peaceful, and which led you to where you wanted to go, would make a great deal of sense.

There has been much debate about ley lines. They have been described as the earth's meridians of energy, which can be tapped just as the meridians of the human body can be used in acupuncture, shiatsu, and magnet therapy. They have been described as lines of magnetic distortion on the magnetic field. They have been assigned powers for both good and evil. It is said that English churches, which were very often built on the sites of much older, pre-Christian, sacred places, are built at junctions of ley lines. Some junctions were beneficial to the buildings that were built there and others were not.

There are many myths and folktales about buildings that collapsed every time they were built. One explanation for this phenomenon is that the doomed structure was being built on a junction of two negative ley lines. But there is a more credible explanation. We know that like poles repel, so if the building stones of these fated structures were from a local seam of rock with a magnetic polarity, perhaps using these rocks on top of the seam created repulsion.

Lines of flux (the concentration of lines of force per unit area, passing from one pole to another) through such a complex and large body as the earth will have localized distortions and eddies within it; this could be a ley line. However, the evidence is inconclusive. If we could harness magnetic influences so that we could float along ley lines, they could become the invisible highways of the future—no pollution, no construction, and no protests. Maybe that is how Merlin was able to travel in Cadair, his magic chair.

Diviners can find ley lines; they claim these are very different from seams of ore. But magnetic influences would naturally concentrate in metallic ore; in fact, magnetism is used to separate out metallic ores in mining processes. Therefore, the claim that the diviner is finding a ley line and not a deep seam of metallic ore does need further investigation.

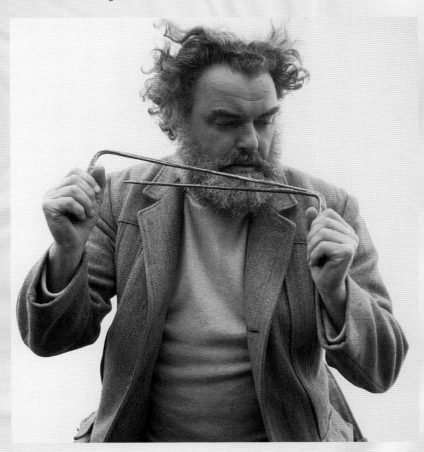

Diviners can locate ley lines and sources of water. Here Cornish diviner Hamish Miller uses his metal rods to scan the earth.

✳ Magnetism and dreams

Dreams of flying are relatively common, and may be explained in a number of ways. In the context of magnet therapy, this ability to soar above the earth may be explained in terms of attraction and repulsion.

We all dream, even if we are not aware of our dreams when we wake up. We are also all subject to magnetic influences, even if we are not aware of this. So there is some kind of connection between dreaming and magnetism: both are part of all our lives, both are largely unconscious, and both are barely understood. So let us look at the possibility that our dreams reflect a long-lost ability to understand and

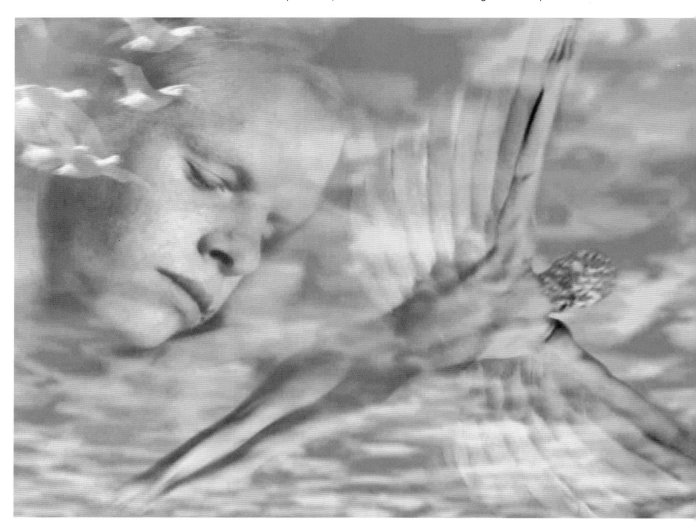

even control magnetic forces. Perhaps dreams that involve attraction by some unseen force—being swept up and pulled toward another person or place—are mimicking the forces of magnetic attraction.

FLYING DREAMS

The complexity of the energy processes that govern our existence surpasses our present understanding, but maybe in flying dreams we allow ourselves to interact with this unseen force and use it to move around. There are common themes in dreams of flying: in some, the dreamer is high above the ground; in others, the dreamer can hardly get off the ground. Flying dreams could be about ambition: when we are flying high, we are achieving our ambitions; when we cannot get very far, we are being frustrated. Perhaps it is the so-called astral body that is escaping the physical body, which would explain the feelings of exultation and freedom that often accompany flying dreams.

We could look at flying dreams in terms of the repulsion and attraction effects of magnets. We feel held down to the earth when we are disengaged from the natural earth—we are opposite to the earth and ruled by the natural law that says unlike poles attract. In another situation, we feel able to fly above the earth because we are at one with it—like poles repel. Perhaps when we dream of being bound to the earth and unable to fly high above it, our dream is trying to tell us to become more natural.

MAGNETIC IMAGES

The images in our dreams, and even our everyday language, indicate our unconscious knowledge of how all-pervading magnetism is. We speak and dream of attractions, unseen forces that pull people together, and of unexplained forces that bind people and events to each other. Myths of flying carpets, of Merlin's Cadair, our own dreams of flying, all point toward the possibility that at some time in ancient history, humankind, or at least a few "wizards," had a greater understanding and even control over natural magnetic forces than we have today, and were able to use them to their own ends. May be an individual who has persistent dreams of flying was one of these people in a past life.

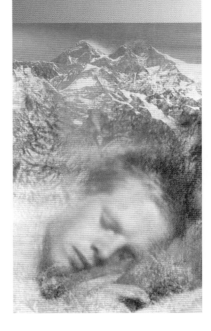

MAGNETIC ATTRACTION

When we dream of being drawn toward some distant mountain, this could be interpreted as some very ancient "memory" of a long-lost human ability to navigate by knowing the location of a particular mountain rich in magnetic lodestone or metallic ore. The idea has been promulgated that our ancient forebears had magnetized material in the nasal cavity and this was some form of natural navigational aid. The dreams of being attracted to a distant mountain could also be a throwback to this ancient heritage.

✳ Magnets and flower remedies

POSSIBLE CONFLICT

Keep magnets away from flower remedies. They are not as delicate as homeopathic remedies but they could be modified by a strong magnetic field that is kept too close to them.

The flower remedy Aspen is given to those who are fearful and anxious. The aspen is a delicate tree, with silvery, quivering leaves—its signature matches the individuals it treats.

Flower remedies are not like other medicines. They do not contain active chemicals or possess pharmaceutical properties. They are best described as a sort of liquid energy, a vibrational medicine that brings about benefits by influencing each person's individual life force.

Flowers, plants, and trees can reflect physical, emotional, or spiritual problems and states. Each flower has its own signature—for example, Eyebright, a blue flower with a yellow center, looks like an eye and is said to help treat eye problems—and its own personality; Clematis, a wistful, clinging plant, is for quiet, dreamy people who are wrapped up in their own thoughts and fantasies. Flower essences can therefore be seen to work on our own subtle vibrational energy (the chi, qi, or life force that has been mentioned previously) to correct physical, emotional, and spiritual problems, and restore a sense of calm and contentment. Because they work on more mental levels than most forms of therapy, the combination of magnet therapy to treat physical symptoms and flower remedies to treat emotional and mental symptoms is a very successful treatment.

COMBINATIONS

In all these cases, magnets should be left in place until relief is obtained. If in doubt, consult your therapist. All flower remedies should be taken internally—they can be dropped on or under the tongue.

For anxiety: Agrimony and 600–800 gauss magnets on St36, Sp6 (if not pregnant), UB11, UB16.

For fear: Aspen, Mimulus, or Rock Rose and 600–800 gauss magnets on St36, Sp6 (if not pregnant), UB11, UB16.

For exhaustion: Olive and 600–800 gauss magnets on Sp6, LI4 (both sides).

For shock: Star of Bethlehem and 600–800 gauss magnets on LI4, Ht7, and Lu1 (both sides). This should be combined with warmth, rest, and fresh air.

For stress: 600–800 gauss magnets on P6 (both sides) on the inside of the wrist between the two blood vessels and about 2–3 inches (5–7 cm)—depending on the size of the arm—from the wrist crease, toward the elbow; B11 and B16 (both sides), between the spine and the shoulder blade, one at the top of the shoulder blade and the other at the bottom. It is often advisable to use doses of Rescue Remedy as a prelude to all the treatments suggested for dealing with stress.

TREATING THE WHOLE PERSON

A human being is an interconnected combination of physical, mental, emotional, and spiritual aspects. We cannot separate one aspect from another, without affecting the other parts of the whole. So it makes sense that ill-health or dis-ease needs a combination of treatments that will improve the well-being of all aspects of the whole person—the spiritual and emotional realms, as well as the physical.

✳ | Magnets and homeopathy

Homeopathy is the treatment of disease with substances that would, in a healthy person, elicit the symptoms of that disease. If we think of health as a state of "ease," both mentally and physically, then illness can be said to be a state of "dis-ease." Homeopathy works with the idea that we all have an innate ability to overcome "dis-ease." The energy, or vitality, that we have within us enables us to grow, repair damaged tissue, respond to different stresses, and generally function with a sense of well-being. We start to produce symptoms—the expression of our "disease"—when we start to feel undue stress.

If we give the appropriate homeopathic remedy in this case, then the body's natural healing energy is stimulated and the body can once again restore itself to balance. Homeopathic remedies allow the body to heal itself, without any of the harmful effects that can come from the use of conventional drugs—they can also make you less susceptible to diseases in the future.

Aconite growing in the wild. As a homeopathic remedy, aconite is useful for treating shock and fevers.

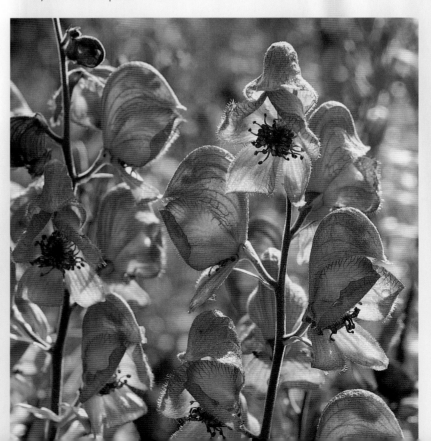

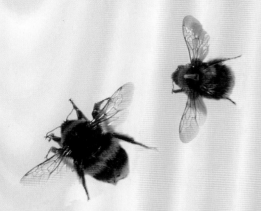

Homeopathy works holistically, and treats the mind, body, and spirit as a whole. Homeopathic remedies work on the principle of like cures like; for example, bees are used to make Apis, which is used to treat bites and stings.

Taking homeopathic remedies should not conflict with any form of magnet therapy; in fact it will enhance the therapeutic activity of the remedies. As the homeopathic remedy kicks into action, the magnets will speed up the flow of body fluids and energy that carry out the corrective action.

Homeopathy can take some time to work when a condition is chronic, and noticeable improvement can take a very long time. Magnet therapy helps to relieve symptoms in the short term, while the patient is waiting for the longer-term benefits of homeopathic treatment.

COMBINATIONS

If taking a remedy for a digestive disorder, use small 600–800 gauss magnets on St36 and LI4 and keep these in place for seven to ten days. If your remedy is for breathing problems, use small 600–800 gauss magnets on LU1, LU9, and SI11. If the remedy is to aid recovery from injury, use magnets and magnetic bandages as described for sports injuries (see pages 60–61). If you are being treated for stress-related problems, then use magnets on the same points used in conjunction with flower remedies for stress (see page 85). With all of the above, keep the magnets in place until relief is obtained. Consult your therapist for more information.

Combining homeopathic remedies with flower remedies, physical therapy, and magnets can speed up the recovery; however, there are a few cautions: do not take your homeopathic remedy at the same time as the flower remedy, and store your magnets well away from flower and homeopathic remedies.

✳ Magnets and shiatsu

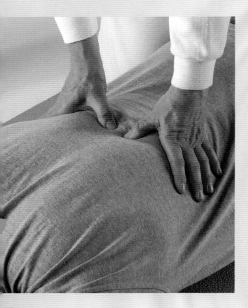

The more vigorous stimulation of acupuncture points occurs during a full-body shiatsu massage, which can also be combined with magnet therapy.

In shiatsu, the practitioner applies various levels of pressure at points along the meridians in order to encourage a balanced and easy flow of energy around the body. Some gentle stretching and easy manipulation may also be involved. There are several styles of shiatsu, but all follow the same general principles. During shiatsu treatments the patient is usually fully clothed, preferably in a tracksuit or other loose clothing, and lies flat on the floor; in conditions where this is difficult for the patient, the treatment can be given with the patient seated. Shiatsu is normally given as a full-body treatment, so it is a great therapy to combine with the more localized and site-specific treatment with magnets. Just as there is a total integration between the physical, emotional, and spiritual bodies, so there is a complete integration of all parts of the physical body. Each organ influences every other organ, each function of the system influences the complete system. So the use of whole-body treatments makes very good sense.

The effect of a full-body treatment, combined with the relaxation and balancing of energy that comes from a good shiatsu session, and the continuous supply of magnetic energy that can be applied to specific points or damaged areas, all work together to give a total effect that is greater than the sum of its parts. If you add flower remedies, meditation, and yoga to these treatments, then you will be following a good holistic program.

A good shiatsu practitioner will be able to advise you on the best places to fix small magnets for your particular condition between full-body treatments. The low cost of small spot magnets and their wide availability means that this is a simple thing to do for yourself. Between treatments, apply 600–800 gauss magnets to the acupressure points. This will enhance the treatments by providing a slow-release stimulation of the point. In cases of sprain or damage to ligaments, you can use bandages or supports that have magnets built into them. Your shiatsu practitioner may be able to obtain these for you or tell you where to buy them.

If your practitioner does not give this advice, remember that knowing where your "ouch points" are can be useful. An "ouch point" is just what it sounds like— when pressure is applied, the recipient says "ouch" as he or she experiences pain. This is a potentially useful point. Apply a small 600–800 gauss magnet or wrap the area with a magnetic bandage to improve the speed of recovery.

CASE STUDY 3

A 52-year-old man came to the shiatsu clinic with a recurring pain and discomfort in his right knee. The usual questions were asked and notes were made on his medical history, diet, stress levels, and whether there were any old injuries. The patient could not remember any specific injury to the painful knee but had played rugby until he was 30 years old. A full shiatsu treatment session proved very useful to the patient, enabling him to relax physically. This provided the practitioner with an insight into his condition and the energy flows of various meridians. Liver energy was blocked off to a degree and the previous conversation had suggested that the patient's alcohol consumption was rather too high.

After the second full shiatsu session, the patient used a magnetic knee-support bandage around the right knee and small spot 600–800 gauss magnets were applied on the points noted by the shiatsu practitioner as being most painful when pressure was applied. (These points will vary from patient to patient, even if they all have painful right knees, because the points are chosen to improve overall energy flows in that unique patient at that time: we will not indicate which points were used in this specific case.)

The magnets were replaced after each shiatsu session, the first three being given on a weekly basis and then two more following at three-week intervals. After the fifth session, the patient was advised to wait a month and then call the clinic. The call indicated that there were no further problems with the knee but the patient did request monthly maintenance sessions.

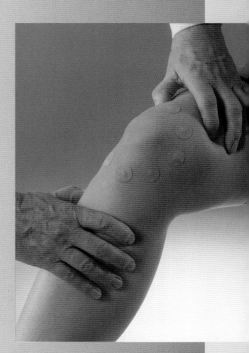

Acupuncture points can be stimulated initially during a shiatsu session to ease pain. Magnets are applied later.

✳ Acupuncture and magnets

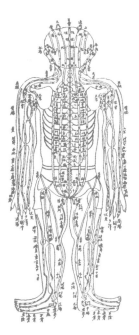

The location of the correct acupuncture points for an individual is a complex process.

LIMITATIONS

It is not practical to stick magnets on many of the acupuncture points. Folds in the elbows, for example, can have a needle in for a 20-minute period, but a magnet will not remain in place if the joint is flexed a few times.

Acupuncture has evolved over about 6,000 years. The first recorded evidence for the therapeutic application of needles to specific points on the body is in a series of Chinese texts written between about 300–100 BCE. It has been said that the origins of acupuncture lay in the observation that soldiers who were suffering from some form of ill-health seemed to recover from their condition after receiving slight puncture wounds in the course of a battle, or during training.

Taoist philosophers discovered that there are pathways of energy that flow around the body; these link together to form a continous flow of life energy—chi or qi. Ill health was thought to be caused by imbalances in the harmonious flow of this energy, imbalances caused by disruptions to the dynamic relationship between yin and yang within that energy. In order to further explain and understand these imbalances, the energy was described in the context of the five elements, or five stages of transformation (see pages 96–103).

Many methods have been used to restore energy balance, but acupuncture has been one of the most enduring and successful. The Chinese developed the system to use over 600 points on the body, in various combinations, to treat a huge variety of conditions. Putting a needle into a person is not difficult, but working out the particular combination of points required to treat the unique condition of an individual human being, while taking into account the interwoven complexity of the effect that ill health has on various parts of the body, and the personal reactions of the individual in question, does require an expert practitioner.

Many of the acupuncture points can be used in magnet therapy, apart from the ones mentioned in the warning box above. It is worth visiting an acupuncture therapist before you start self-help magnet therapy, just to know where the exact points are.

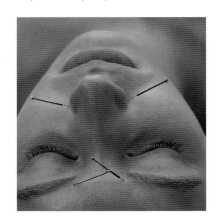

Acupuncture needles can alarm some people. In such cases, acupuncture points can be treated with small magnets.

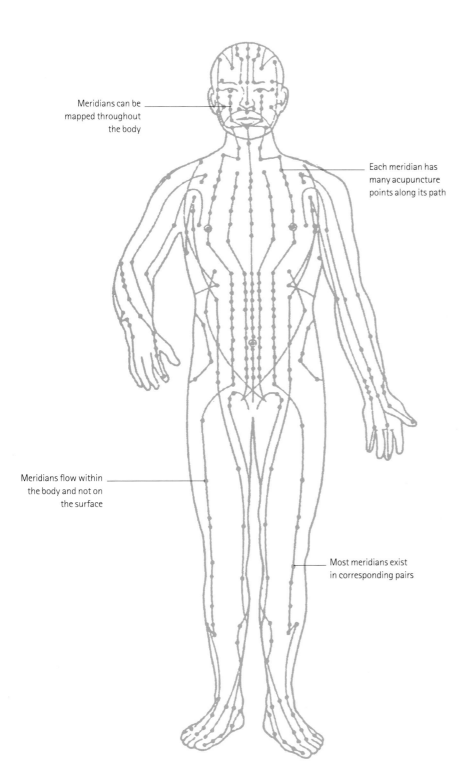

Meridians can be mapped throughout the body

Each meridian has many acupuncture points along its path

Meridians flow within the body and not on the surface

Most meridians exist in corresponding pairs

COMBINING TREATMENTS

If various therapies are combined, it is impossible to know which therapy is most beneficial. For some people this may present a problem. However, the object of treatment is to improve the well-being of the recipient, not to test which is the best therapy. In clinical trials, it may be important to study each therapy in isolation, but for general healthcare, the quickest, most effective improvement is all that matters. The total effect of combined treatments is often greater than the sum of the parts, so trying many treatments may have the desired effect—a speedy recovery and improved resilience.

The meridians are a complex map throughout the body, forming the pathways along which our internal energy flows. Each individual will have different energy balances and imbalances.

✳ Experimenting with magnetism

Playing around with magnets is the best way to learn about their properties. Always consult a practitioner before attempting any treatment with magnets yourself.

Children's kits of magnets come with instructions for simple experiments. The advantage, apart from the relatively low cost, of these kits is that they almost always have the poles marked—usually as north, meaning north-seeking, and south meaning south-seeking. The disadvantage is that they do not indicate the strength of the magnets. You can determine magnets' relative strength by testing their ability to pick up objects of different weights.

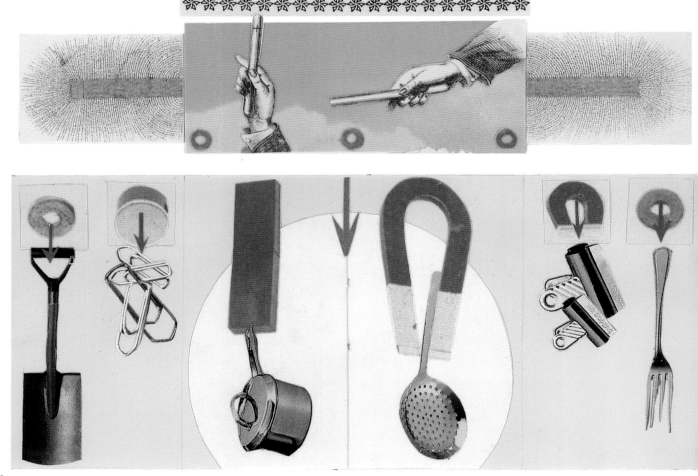

SIMPLE EXPERIMENTS

Here is a list of simple but interesting experiments:

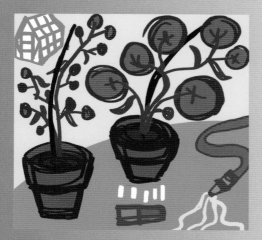

In the greenhouse, stand some tomato plants on magnets and see if they provide a better crop than those without magnets. Water some with magnetized water and see if they grow more or larger fruit than those given ordinary water.

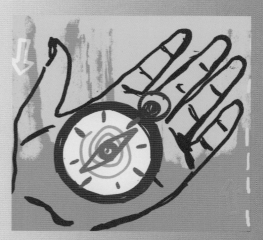

Try to find ley lines. Walk along the line with a compass and see if the needle is always constant in its direction or whether it makes unexplained deviations.

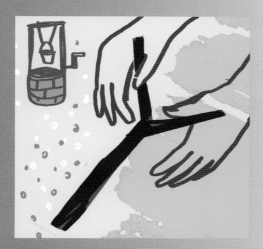

Use divining twigs and rods. Focus your mind on magnetic forces and see if you can get the rods to move.

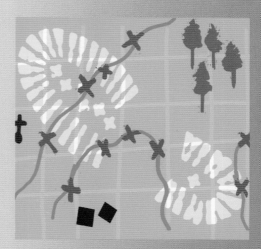

Walk back and forth over a large area and make a map of where the deviations of the compass or the movement of the divining rods occur.

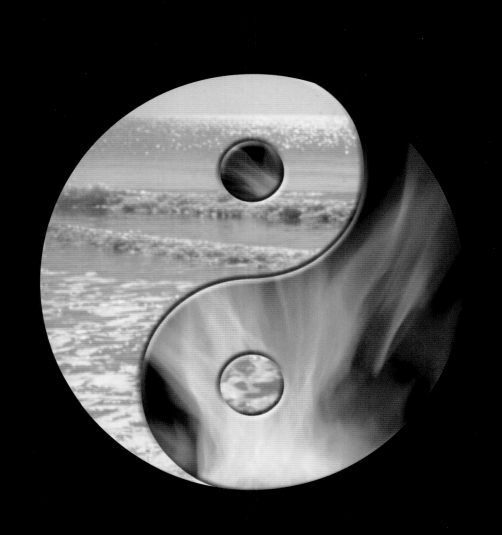

✳ | Chapter five

Applying the theory This section begins with an overview of the five transformations theory and the yin and yang energies. These are vital to the understanding of the meridians, which, in turn, are very important to the practice of magnet therapy and the use of acupuncture points. There are also 14 charts showing the position of the meridians discussed in the book, and a list of acupuncture points under each meridian, with the symptoms that they treat.

The elements of Chinese philosophy

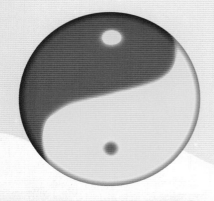

The properties of yin and yang are mutable and everchanging. They often meld into each other, making them difficult to define.

It is important to understand the background behind acupuncture and shiatsu because it informs much of the theory that lies behind magnet therapy. The elements of yin and yang are vital to both these therapies, and to the practice of magnet therapy itself.

Chinese medical texts state that "every object or phenomenon in the universe consists of two opposite aspects, namely, yin and yang, which are at once in conflict and in interdependence." For a moment, think of yin as a pot of red paint and yang as a pot of yellow paint. If we take a small part of yin (red) and add it to some yang (yellow), the result is a third color. By adding various amounts of red to various amounts of yellow, we can get an infinite number of other colors. Now think of yin and yang as entities in their own right, rather than different colored paints: a small part of one added to part of the other produces a third entity, and so on. This can be done an infinite number of times—the Chinese ancients referred to this infinite number as the "ten thousand things," because they did not have a word for "infinite," or a number to represent that amount.

The concept of yin and yang can also be thought of as ethereal and material, or nonphysical and physical. In this way, the combination of parts of each to make a third entity begins to make more sense. If we consider human beings to be a particular combination of a certain amount of yin and a certain amount of yang, then it is an easy step to see that a slight adjustment in this mixture would lead to a male and another small adjustment would lead to a female. Just as physical matter can be of a differing density, so we can have different degrees of intensity of yin and yang within any particular combination. A pebble on the beach is not the same size as a mountain; similarly, the total sum of yin and yang within any object is infinitely variable, and within that given total the ratio of yin to yang can also be infinitely variable. The ratio of yin to yang within any entity is also not static and is everchanging and flowing within the limits imposed on it by that entity. For example, an inanimate object can be defined as an object that has the ratio of yin and yang static within it, but the more variable the ratio of yin and yang—within the limits of the nature of the entity—the more mobility that entity has.

The reason that the traditional yin/yang symbol is drawn the way it is is to show that yin can become yang—and of course yang can become yin—and also that within yin there is some yang—and within yang there is some yin. The whole thing is flowing and changing within its own particular limitations. To describe this in terms of human emotions, anger can become fear, while fear can easily become anger, but there is a limit to the amount of fear and anger any particular individual can cope with. The actual amount varies from person to person but the mix between fear and anger ebbs and flows within that person's limits. There is also a particular combination of yin and yang within each human, which should be near equal in its balance. Ancient Chinese scholars used the elements of water and fire to symbolize the basic properties of yin and yang, with yin as water and yang as fire. Therefore, it can be seen that the properties of yin are coldness, dampness, and downward direction (like a waterfall), while the properties of yang are heat, brightness, and upward direction (like a flame).

THE FIVE TRANSFORMATIONS

The five transformations are used to record and communicate any variations and fluctuations in the rhythm of our overall cycle at any particular time. These five transformations are sometimes called the five elements but, because they are more like stages of transformation, and we can move from one to another, the name "element" can sometimes be misleading, as it has connotations of fixed and immutable characteristics. The five stages in a cycle of transformation are called fire, earth, metal (sometimes called air), water, and wood. (Metal is used here in the Old English sense—anything that comes from the earth is called metal; a paved road is sometimes still called a metalled road.) A particular person can be predominantly wood but an organ or a function within that same person could be predominantly water. We can equally say that a person is a "fire" person but that their heart is metal, and vice versa.

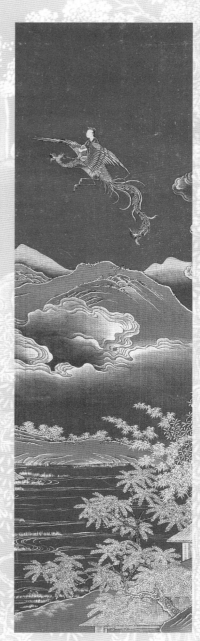

The five stages in the Ancient Chinese cycle of transformation—fire, earth, metal, water, and wood—are depicted in this painting.

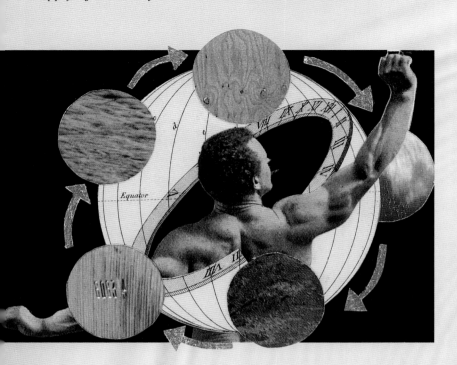

The theory of the five elements or five transformations is the cornerstone philosophy of traditional Chinese medicine.

The concept of the five transformations is simple in outline and complex in detail. The simple concept is that they are set at intervals around a circle and movement can be around that circle, from one place to the next. On a more complex level, the five stages are also symbolic: they are a way of putting into writing the observations and perceptions gained over thousands of years by the Chinese ancients. For example, a metal personality is rigid, unable to flex and bend; such a personality can be overcome with grief because they do not allow themselves to show it and it overwhelms them in a destructive manner. A "fire" person can easily burn out their body and heart by being too emotionally fragile and trying to seek enjoyment in every moment of their lives. The five transformations are all contained within the body and are all interdependent. They are all also in a state of constant motion and change. When all is in balance within the body, the flow from one stage of transformation to the next occurs easily and naturally: this is called the interpromoting relationship. When all is in harmony, this goes round the circle from wood, to fire, to earth, to metal, to water, and then back to wood.

When there is an imbalance of energy damaging reactions take place. When this causes a stage to get missed out, then this is called the overacting relationship; if the imbalance causes the energies to try to run in an opposite direction, then this is called a counteracting relationship. The effect of energy imbalances often has multiple results, and excess and insufficiency can exist at the same time within the same person. For example, if wood is in excess then it overacts on earth and it can counteract on metal, throwing the whole system out of balance. This relationship between the stages of a cycle can be used to explain why a disease may spread or change into something different within the body. How many people each year make regular visits to the general practitioner with a different illness each time? It is probable that 20 percent of the patients on one doctor's register will take up 80 percent of surgery time, with recurring complaints that have differing symptoms.

If we apply the five transformations theory to this situation, we can see that the excess or insufficiency has moved to a different part of the cycle, and that although the physical symptoms may seem to be different, it is really the same basic imbalance that causes the problems. If the complex changes in a disease are analyzed in the context of the five transformations theory, then they all come under four conditions:

- **overacting**
- **counteracting**
- **mother affecting son**
- **son affecting mother**

For example, pulmonary disease may in some cases be caused by heart malfunction; in the five transformations theory this is known as fire overacting on metal. If the liver was the prime cause, then wood would be counteracting on metal. If you observe the direction of energy flow during the stages of transformation it can be seen that, for example, metal comes from earth and so earth is said to be the "mother" of metal. Thus, we can use a "mother" point—in this case, acupuncture point Liver 9—to foster the transformation to metal. If a patient lacked cohesion, i.e., was too flexible, then the use of L9 (the earth point that is the mother of metal) to feed the metal characteristic would be of help to that patient. The "son" point of metal is acupuncture point Liver 5. Water comes from metal (think of condensation forming on cold metal) so it is necessary to reduce the energy in the metal characteristic of the patient because they are too rigid; in this case the "son" point L5 should be stimulated.

Many hundreds of years of experience have led to this concept of the five transformations being of great use in diagnostic work. For example, a person who has a bitter taste in the mouth and a florid (hot) complexion should be checked over for a weakness or excess in the heart. Emotional responses to any energy imbalances can also manifest themselves. The emotional condition can indicate what the energy problems are that are affecting physical health and where this is occurring. Everything is interdependent and cause and effect are interchangeable.

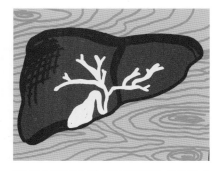

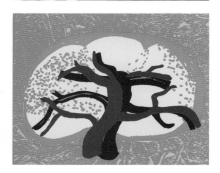

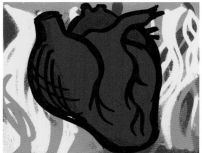

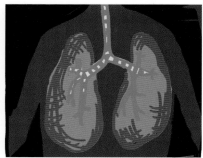

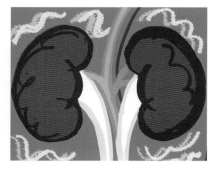

Each of the five transformations can affect the main organs in the body—liver, heart, spleen, lungs, and kidneys. Our emotional state can also change the ways these function.

HOW EMOTIONS AFFECT THE FIVE TRANSFORMATIONS

- Anger is related to the liver and, in turn, this affects the strength of the muscles; the liver can also be associated with depression. The reverse of this can be seen when a depressive patient may start to suffer from a deterioration in the liver's function.
- Excessive and inappropriate happiness is associated with heart and circulation problems. Melancholia can also follow, or lead to, heart and circulatory disorders.
- The spleen is related to excessive sympathy, anxiety, and lifeless flesh.
- The lungs are related to grief, sadness, and a deterioration in the condition of the skin and hair.
- The kidneys are connected to fear, withdrawal from responsibilities, and swelling of the joints.

These connections show that if we can improve the emotional well-being of a patient, then we are helping them work on the organ dysfunction and the surface symptoms they are suffering from.

THE FIVE TRANSFORMATIONS IN MAGNET THERAPY

In magnet therapy it is the practice to find, by observation, questioning, and touch, where the likely areas of excess and depletion are in the patient. Then north-seeking magnetic poles are used against the depleted points and south-seeking magnetic poles are used against the points of excess. Advice is given to patients so they can adjust the flows of energy around the body by themselves between sessions. The aim is to get the body to rebalance itself. A "cure" is not imposed on the body: it is preferable to allow the body to work through its natural mechanisms on its own to find its true point of balance. However, there are times when the level of pain or disability is so great that a patient cannot function properly and the

CLASSICAL ACUPUNCTURE POINTS

In classical acupuncture the stages of transformation are given to specific acupuncture points as follows:

 WOOD   Lung 1, Spleen 1, Heart 9, Kidney 1, Pericardium 9, Liver 1, Large Intestine 3, Stomach 43, Small Intestine 3, Bladder 65, Triple Heater 3, Gall Bladder 41.

 FIRE   Lung 10, Spleen 2, Heart 8, Kidney 2, Pericardium 8, Liver 2, Large Intestine 5, Stomach 41, Small Intestine 5, Bladder 60, Triple Heater 6, Gall Bladder 38.

 EARTH   Lung 9, Spleen 3, Heart 7, Kidney 6, Pericardium 7, Liver 3, Large Intestine 1, Stomach 36, Small Intestine 8, Bladder 54, Triple Heater 10, Gall Bladder 34.

 METAL   Lung 8, Spleen 5, Heart 4, Kidney 7, Pericardium 5, Liver 4, Large Intestine 1, Stomach 45, Small Intestine 1, Bladder 67, Triple Heater 1, Gall Bladder 44.

 WATER   Lung 5, Spleen 9, Heart 3, Kidney 10, Pericardium 3, Liver 8, Large Intestine 2, Stomach 44, Small Intestine 2, Bladder 66, Triple Heater 2, Gall Bladder 43.

quality of life is reduced to an unacceptable degree. Natural medicines usually take some time to achieve the long-lasting rebalancing that is needed for a healthy body—this is a cumulative effect, which gradually improves the illness in question. In these cases, it is necessary for patients to use chemical aids to stabilize their position. Also, if physical manipulation is used to "push" some postural error back into place, then the patient must be shown the exercises that will retrain the body to hold this correct posture, and therefore prevent a recurrence of the bad one. The five transformation stages and the overall cycle can help to guide the patient toward a restoration of a natural, gentle, flowing cycle of energy, and then a complete return to good health.

- Wood is burned by fire to produce ash (earth). Air/earth produce water.
- Water enables wood to grow.
- Air is sometimes called metal. Air condenses on cold metal to form water.
- Metal in Old English is any material dug from the ground (earth).
- Metal controls wood—wood controls earth—earth controls water.

THE FIVE TRANSFORMATIONS

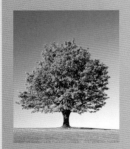 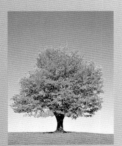 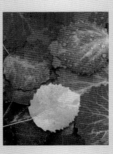 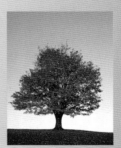 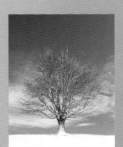

PERIOD OF WOOD STAGE	PERIOD OF FIRE STAGE	PERIOD OF EARTH STAGE	PERIOD OF METAL STAGE	PERIOD OF WATER STAGE
Spring 73 days	*Summer 73 days*	*Late summer 73 days*	*Autumn 73 days*	*Winter 73 days*
Soul	*Spirit*	*Ideas*	*Animal spirit*	*Will power*
Sour taste	*Bitter taste*	*Sweet taste*	*Pungent taste*	*Salty taste*
Liver/Gall Bladder	*Heart/Small Intestine*	*Spleen/stomach*	*Lung/Large Intestine*	*Kidney/Bladder*
Green	*Red*	*Yellow*	*White*	*Black*
Muscles	*Blood vessels*	*Flesh*	*Skin and hair*	*Bones/marrow*

The start of the year is February 21 in the UK and US.

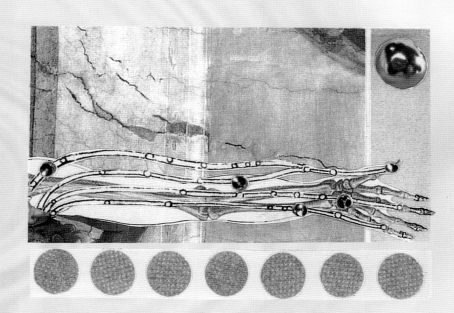

Magnets applied to acupuncture points act in a less invasive way than a needle, and provide gentle pressure and slowly released energy.

USING MAGNETISM

A magnet placed on an acupuncture point acts as a slow-release acupuncture needle treatment. It is a good alternative to acupuncture for those who are afraid of needles or dislike the pain of acupuncture.

The study of acupuncture and all the points—what they can be used for, the best times to use them, the correct combination of points, etc—is an extremely complex subject and beyond the scope of this book. We will look at some basic ways you can use small magnets stuck to selected points to improve well-being and speed up recovery from injury and illness.

Each individual is different, so it is not possible to quantify the relative amounts of energy in any part of the system at any time. The condition of each organ and the overall condition of the body will affect this and change with the time of day and the season.

Because energy flows in a continuous cycle around all the organs, a holistic approach is vital; we cannot consider the heart in isolation from the lungs, or any other part of the body, because all parts are linked together.

✳ | The meridians

SHIATSU AND YOGA

Shiatsu practitioners determine where on the meridians energy is blocked, stagnant, or depleted. They then use pressure, manipulation, and massage techniques to get the energy flowing again. Yoga postures are designed to stretch and open up the meridians, thus preventing blockages, stagnation, and depletion.

A sequence of yoga positions is designed to open up the meridian channels, freeing any blocked energy that may be caught there.

Energy flows around the body along meridians that are linked together to form a continuous loop. At certain points it is possible to access this energy flow. These are the acupuncture points, called *tsubos* in Japanese shiatsu. By attaching small magnets to the correct point, we can affect the flow of energy and thereby affect the well-being of the body. There is always energy in all parts of the system, but the proportion of the total will vary with one's state of health, the time of day, and the period of the year. The flows of energy around the body along the meridians follow a 24-hour cycle. Each type of energy has a specific period when it predominates.

All energy contains complementary forces of both yin and yang, but meridians are classified as yin or yang depending on which predominates. Do remember that being predominantly yin does not mean that yang is excluded.

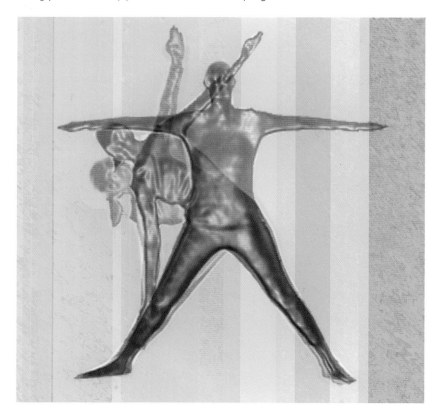

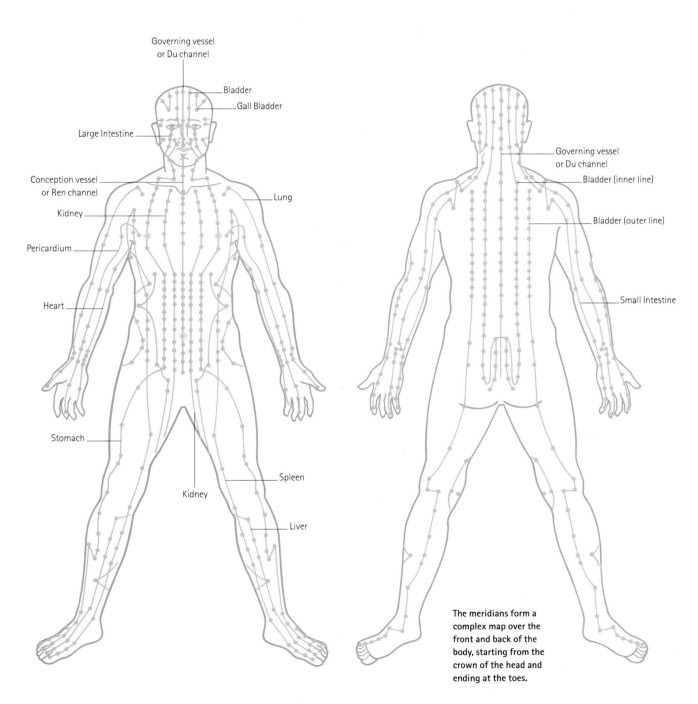

Governing vessel
or Du channel

Bladder

Gall Bladder

Large Intestine

Conception vessel
or Ren channel

Kidney

Pericardium

Heart

Stomach

Kidney

Spleen

Liver

Lung

Governing vessel
or Du channel

Bladder (inner line)

Bladder (outer line)

Small Intestine

The meridians form a
complex map over the
front and back of the
body, starting from the
crown of the head and
ending at the toes.

THE MERIDIANS

MERIDIAN	TIME OF PREDOMINANCE	TYPE	ENERGY PATH
Lung	3 a.m. to 5 a.m.	yin	Liver to Large Intestine
Large Intestine	5 a.m. to 7 a.m.	yang	Lung to Stomach
Stomach	7 a.m. to 9 a.m.	yang	Large Intestine to Spleen
Spleen	9 a.m. to 11 a.m.	yin	Stomach to Heart
Heart	11 a.m. to 1 p.m.	yin	Spleen to Small Intestine
Small Intestine	1 p.m. to 3 p.m.	yang	Heart to Urinary Bladder
Urinary Bladder	3 p.m. to 5 p.m.	yang	Small Intestine to Kidney
Kidney	5 p.m. to 7 p.m.	yin	Urinary Bladder to Pericardium *(Heart Governor, Heart Constrictor)*
Pericardium *(sometimes called Heart Governor or Heart Constrictor or Circulation Sex meridian)*	7 p.m. to 9 p.m.	yin	Kidney to Meridian Triple Heater *(Triple Warmer)*
Triple Heater *(sometimes called Triple Warmer)*	9 p.m. to 11 p.m.	yang	Pericardium to Gall Bladder
Gall Bladder	11 p.m. to 1 a.m.	yang	Triple Heater *(Triple Warmer)* to Liver
Liver	1 a.m. to 3 a.m.	yin	Gall Bladder to Lung

THE EXTRA MERIDIANS

There are several "accepted" extra meridians; the two predominant ones of these are the Governing Vessel, which runs up the center line of the back, and the Conception Vessel, which runs up the center line of the front. These two meridians form their own "loop."

The following list show dates of predominance: the meridians also have seasons of predominance.

February 21 to May 4	**May 5 to July 16**	**July 17 to September 27**	**September 28 to December 9** Lung and	**December 10 to February 20** Kidney
Liver and Gall Bladder	Heart and Small Intestine	Spleen and Stomach	Large Intestine	and Bladder

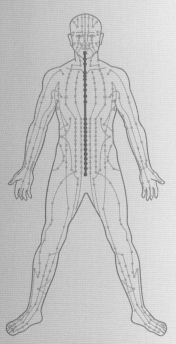

the Ren Channel or
Conception Vessel Meridian

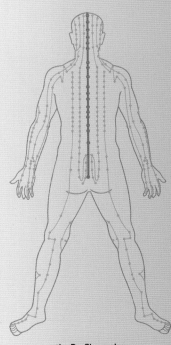

the Du Channel or
Governing Vessel Meridian

MAGNETS AS AN ALTERNATIVE TO ACUPUNCTURE

Small magnets (600–800 gauss) on acupuncture points will stimulate that point and act as a slow-release acupuncture needle treatment. Some acupuncture points are not suitable for magnet therapy because the magnets will not stay in place on creases or folds, such as on the elbow crease or wrist crease. The following charts show the main points used in magnet therapy and the symptoms they treat.

LUNG MERIDIAN

POINT	SYMPTOMS TO BE TREATED
1	cough, asthma, and chest pain
2	coughs, asthma, pain in arm/shoulder and chest
4	pain in arm
6	sore throat, pain in elbow and arm
7	headache, sore throat
8	cough, sore throat, pain in wrist
10	cough, fever

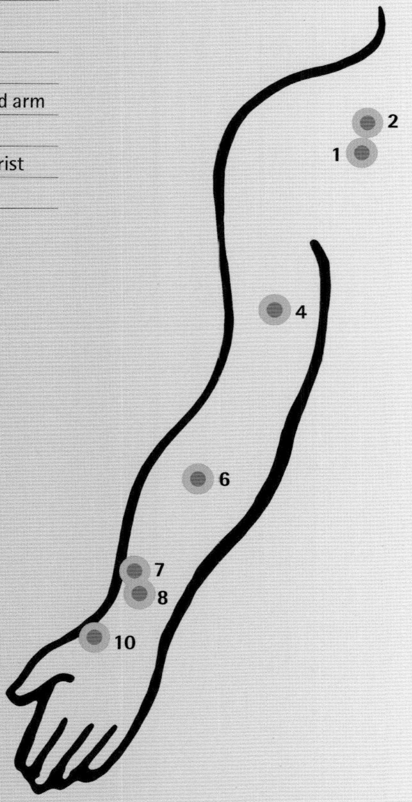

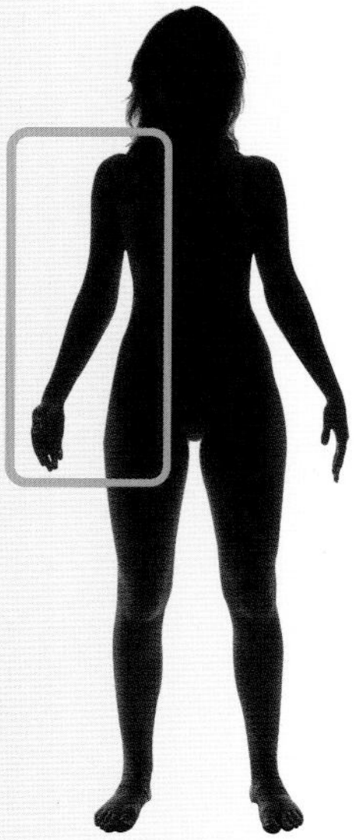

LARGE INTESTINE MERIDIAN

POINT	SYMPTOMS TO BE TREATED
2	toothache, sore throat
4	a general point to use in almost all cases of weakness, headache, pain in eyes, toothache, pain in arms, abdominal pain, constipation
6	aches in hand and arm
7	headache, sore throat, abdominal pain, aches in shoulder and arm
8	abdominal pain, pain in elbow
9	aches in shoulder
10	vomiting, diarrhea, abdominal pain
12	pain or numbness in elbow and arm
14	pain in shoulder and arm
15	pain in shoulder and arm
16	pain in shoulder
17	sore throat, loss of voice
18	cough, asthma, sore throat, loss of voice

STOMACH MERIDIAN

POINT	SYMPTOMS TO BE TREATED
9	sore throat, dizziness, red flushes in face
10	sore throat, asthma
12	cough, sore throat
14	chest pain, cough
15	pain in breast, chest pain
18	chest pain, lactation deficiency
19	abdominal distension, vomiting, gastric pain, possible use in anorexia
20	same as point 19
21	abdominal distension, gastric pain
22	diarrhea, abdominal pain
23	indigestion, restlessness, irritability
24	gastric pain
25	main treatment point for digestive problems, abdominal pain and distention, constipation, diarrhea, irregular menstruation
27	distention of lower abdomen
31	pain in thigh and loss of mobility in leg, muscle wastage
32	pain in lower parts of the leg
34	pain and swelling in the knee
36	a main treatment point for digestive problems, gastric pain, indigestion, abdominal swelling, vomiting, dizziness, aches in leg and knee
38	pain in leg, pain in shoulder
39	pain in leg, ankle, and feet
40	chest pain, headaches, dizziness
41	headache, vertigo, constipation, depression
42	pain and swelling in foot
43	abdominal pain, pain in foot

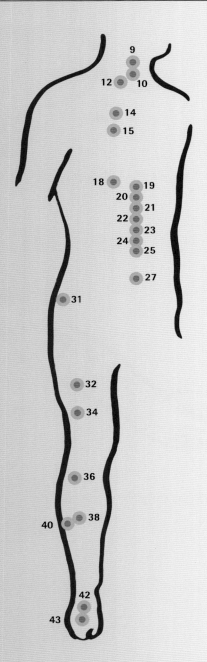

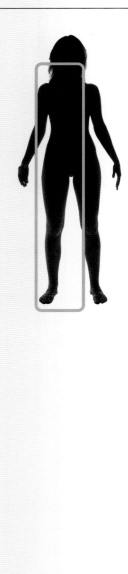

SPLEEN MERIDIAN

POINT	SYMPTOMS TO BE TREATED
2	gastric pain
3	constipation, vomiting, sluggishness
4	abdominal pain
6	Not to be used in pregnancy. A general point for almost all health problems specific to females; also for insomnia, and pain in lower legs and feet
7	abdominal distention, numbness in knee and leg
8	irregular menstruation, anorexia
9	abdominal distention, jaundice, pain in knee
10	pain in knee, pain in thigh, eczema
11	swelling in the groin area, particularly the ligaments in the groin area
15	constipation, pain in lower abdomen
16	constipation, general abdominal pain
21	pain in chest, asthma, general aches and weakness

Note *Spleen points 2–11 run up the inside of the leg.*

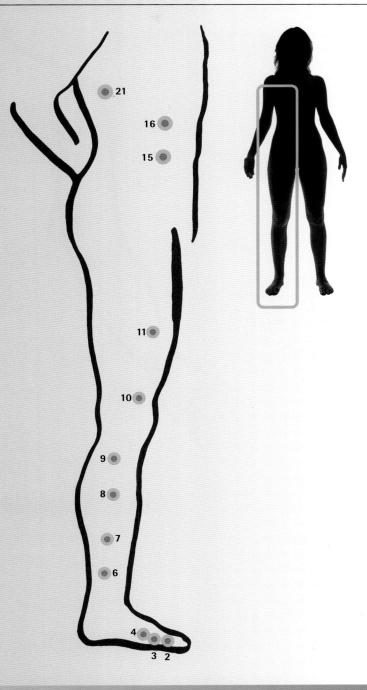

HEART MERIDIAN

POINT	SYMPTOMS TO BE TREATED
1	pain in elbow and arm
2	pain in shoulder and arm
3	cardiac pain, numb feeling in arm, shakes in the hand
4	cardiac pain, sudden loss of voice, convulsions
5	dizziness, blurred vision, sore throat, pain in wrist and arm
6	cardiac pain, hysteria
8	chest pain, palpitation

Note *Heart point 1 is located in the armpit.*

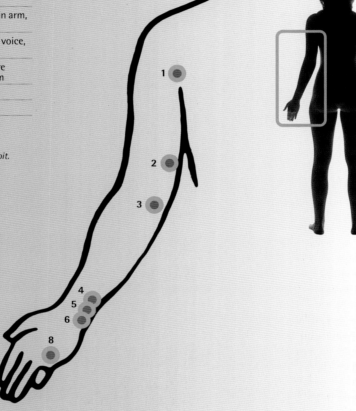

SMALL INTESTINE MERIDIAN

POINT	SYMPTOMS TO BE TREATED
3	headache, stiff neck, eye problems
4	headache, stiff neck, jaundice
7	pain in fingers, stiff neck, mental and emotional upsets
9	pain in shoulder blade, pain in hand and arm
10	pains and weakness in shoulder and arm
11	pain in shoulder blade, lung or breathing problems
12	numbness and aches in upper arms
13	pain and stiffness in shoulder blade
14	stiff neck
15	cough, asthma, pains in upper back
16	sore throat, stiff and painful neck
18	toothache
19	ear problems and pain

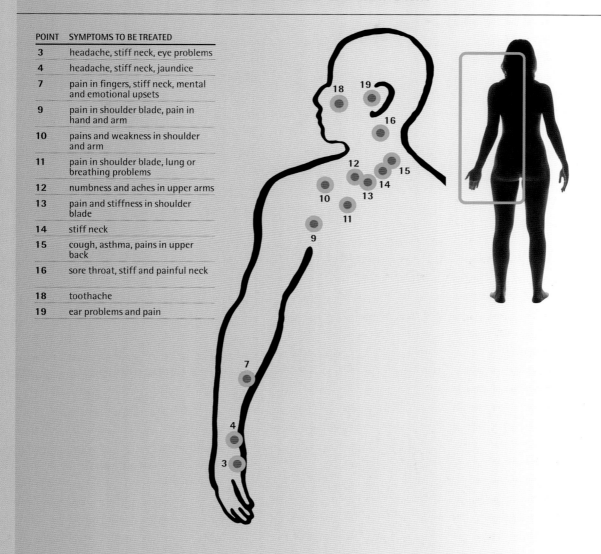

BLADDER MERIDIAN (URINARY BLADDER MERIDIAN)

POINT	SYMPTOMS TO BE TREATED
10	headache, stiff neck, shoulder and back pain
11	cough, fever, headaches, stiff neck
12	common cold, cough, fever, backache
13	a main treatment point for the lungs, coughs, asthma
14	a main treatment point for the pericardium, chest pain, poor circulation
15	a main treatment point for the heart, panic, palpitation, irritability, cough
16	cardiac pain, abdominal pain
17	nausea, difficulty in swallowing, asthma
18	a main treatment point for the liver, jaundice, mental confusion, pain in back, blurred vision
19	a main treatment point for the gall bladder, jaundice, chest pain
20	a main treatment point for the spleen, abdominal distention, nausea, diarrhea, indigestion, pain in back
21	a main treatment point for stomach, chest pain, abdominal distention, nausea, indigestion
22	nausea, indigestion, pain and stiffness in lower back
23	a main treatment point for the kidneys, problems with hearing, backache, weakness in knees, irregular menstruation
24	lower back pain
25	constipation, lower back pain, abdominal pain and distention
26	same as point 25
27	lower abdominal pain
28	a main treatment point for the bladder, constipation, retention of urine, stiff and painful lower back
37	pain in lower back and thigh
39	cramp in leg and foot, pain in lower back

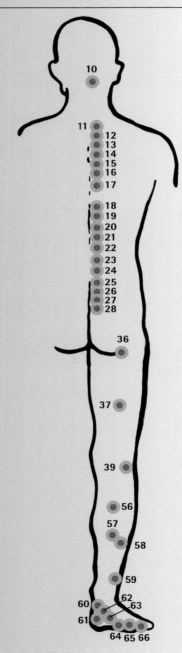

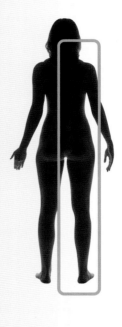

POINT	SYMPTOMS TO BE TREATED
56	pain in leg, hemorrhoids, acute lower back pain
57	constipation, hemorrhoids, lower back pain
58	headache, blurred vision, lumbago, weakness in leg
59	headache, lower back pain
60	spasm and pain in shoulder and arm, backache, pain in heel, headache
61	pain in heel, weakness in legs
63	backache
64	stiff neck, pain in back and legs, headache
65	blurred vision, mental confusion, pain in backs of legs
66	headaches, blurred vision, stiff neck

KIDNEY MERIDIAN

POINT	SYMPTOMS TO BE TREATED
2	pain and swelling in foot
3	toothache, pain in lower back, too frequent micturition (passing urine), sore throat, asthma
8	constipation, irregular menstruation
9	pain in legs, mental pain
11	retention of urine, impotence
13	diarrhea
15	constipation, lower abdominal pain
16	abdominal pain, vomiting, constipation
19	abdominal pain and distention
20	indigestion, nausea, abdominal pain
25	cough, asthma, chest pain
26	cough, asthma, feeling of fullness in chest
27	chest pain, cough, asthma

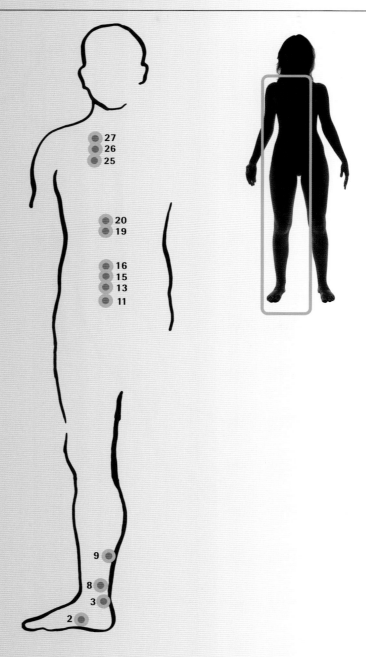

PERICARDIUM MERIDIAN

POINT	SYMPTOMS TO BE TREATED
1	sensation of suffocation within the chest
2	pain in cardiac region, chest pain, cough, pain in upper arm
4	cardiac pain, palpitation
5	pain in arm, gastric pain, vomiting
6	nausea, vomiting, travel sickness, morning sickness
8	fungal infections of hand and foot

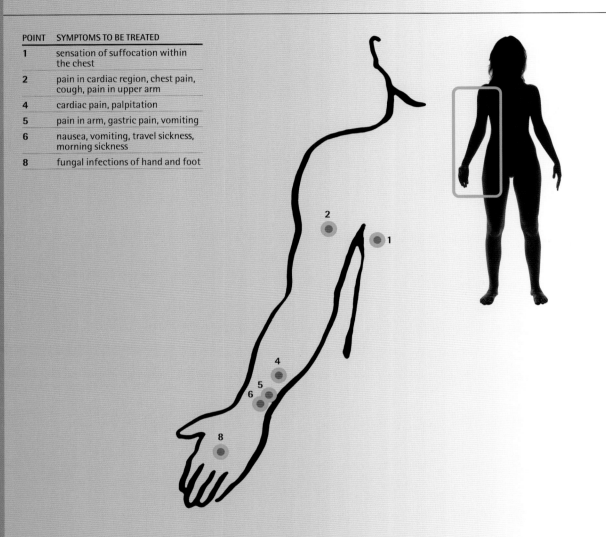

TRIPLE HEATER MERIDIAN (TRIPLE WARMER)

POINT	SYMPTOMS TO BE TREATED
3	hearing and ears, pain in elbow and arm, loss of mobility in fingers
5	pain and loss of movement in fingers, elbow, and arm, pain in face, headaches
6	problems with ears and hearing, constipation, aches in shoulders
8	pain in hand and arm
9	toothache, pain in forearm
11	pain in shoulder and arm
12	stiff and painful neck, pain in arm
13	pain in shoulder and arm
14	pain in arm
15	pain in shoulder and arm, pain with stiffness in neck
16	dizziness, facial swelling, blurred vision, stiff neck
20	toothache, problems with eyes

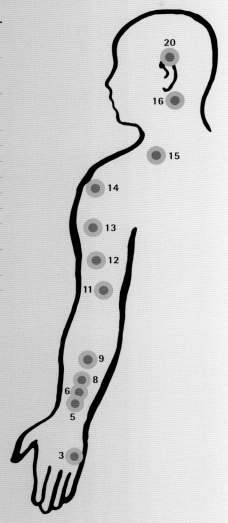

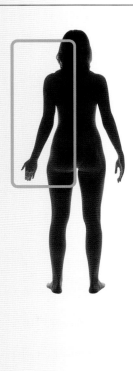

GALL BLADDER MERIDIAN

POINT	SYMPTOMS TO BE TREATED
1	toothache, ear problems
2	headache, ear problems, toothache
3	same as point 2
4	one-sided headache, blurred vision
14	frontal headache, blurred vision
20	headaches, dizziness, pain in shoulders and back, stiff neck
21	stiff neck, pain in shoulder and back, loss of movement in arm and hand
24	a main treatment point for the gall bladder, jaundice, hiccups, nausea
25	abdominal distention, diarrhea, lower back pain
26	lower back pain
27	pain in hip joint and lower back
28	same as point 27
29	pain in lower legs
30	pain in lower back and hip joints
31	hormone or digestive enzyme-production difficulties, period pain, difficulty in digesting foods, pain anywhere in leg or knee
32	numbness and loss of movement in legs
34	pain and swelling in knee
35	knee pain, weakness in foot
36	pain in neck, chest pain
37	pain in knee
38	one-sided headache
40	pain in neck, chest pain, acid regurgitation, pain and swelling in ankles
41	pain and swelling in foot
42	problems with eyes, pain in foot, lack of oxygen reaching the brain
43	blurred vision, pain in face, ear problems, lack of oxygen reaching the brain

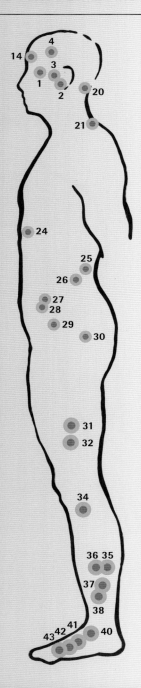

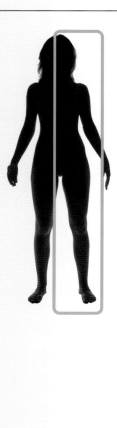

LIVER MERIDIAN

POINT	SYMPTOMS TO BE RELIEVED
2	pain and problems with eyes, headaches, lack of oxygen to brain
3	vertigo, headaches, insomnia
4	retention of urine
5	pain in leg
7	pain in front of knee
9	lower back pain
10	lower abdominal distention
11	pain in thigh and leg
12	hernia
13	a main treatment point for the spleen, indigestion, vomiting, abdominal distention
14	a main treatment point for the liver, chest pain, vomiting

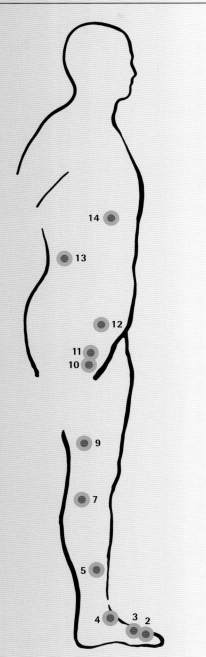
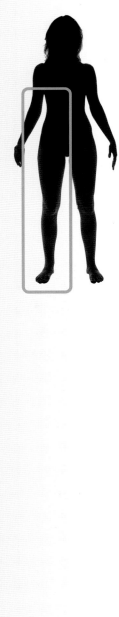

GOVERNING VESSEL MERIDIAN (THE DU CHANNEL)

POINT	SYMPTOMS TO BE TREATED
3	pain in lumbar and sacral area, numbness and loss of mobility in legs
4	stiff back
5	inability to digest food fully, pain and stiffness in lower back
6	jaundice
7	lower back pain
8	gastric problems, lower back pain
9	cough, asthma, jaundice, stiffness in spine
10	stiff neck, cough, asthma
11	anxiety, cardiac pain, stiff back, cough
12	stiffness in lower back, cough, asthma
13	headache
22	headache, blurred vision
24	anxiety, headaches, insomnia, vertigo

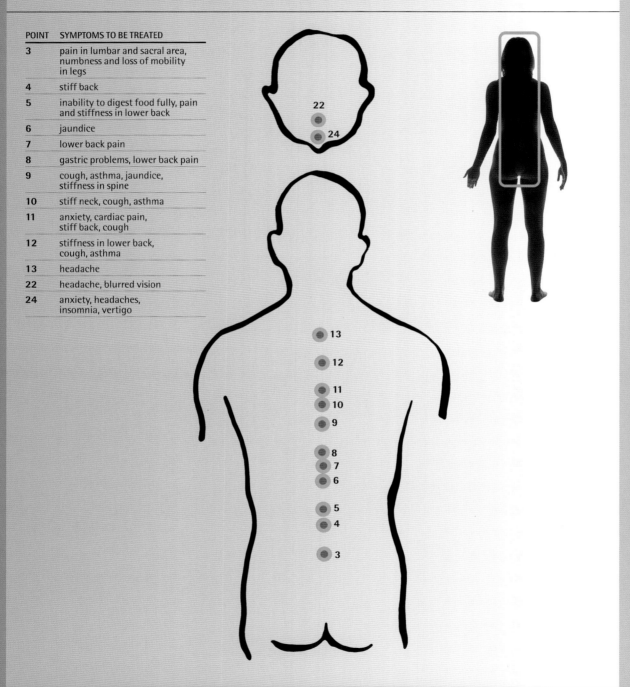

CONCEPTION VESSEL MERIDIAN (THE REN CHANNEL)

POINT	SYMPTOMS TO BE TREATED
3	a main treatment point for the bladder, all disorders of the bladder, pain in lower abdomen
4	pain in lower abdomen, diarrhea
5	abdominal pain
6	constipation, abdominal pain
7	pain around the area of the umbilicus
9	abdominal pain
10	gastric pain, inability to digest food fully
11	gastric pain, some reports of use in anorexia
12	a main treatment point for the stomach, inability to digest food fully, abdominal pain, gastric pain
14	a main treatment point for the heart, chest pain, difficulty in swallowing, nausea, palpitations
15	chest pain
16	difficulty in swallowing
17	a main treatment point for pericardium and circulation, hiccups, chest pain
18	cough, chest pain
19	same as point 18
20	same as point 18
21	same as point 18
22	sore throat, cough, loss of voice

✳ | Glossary

acupoint – *the point along a meridian at which the life force (chi or qi) is thought to be accessible. Acupoints are stimulated by the insertion of needles or by acupressure.*

aura – *every person, animal, and plant is said to have a visible aura, or magnetic field. The aura is said to indicate the state of a person's physical, mental, emotional, and spiritual health.*

channel – see *meridians.*

complementary – *the term used to describe alternative forms of medical treatment, emphasizing the fact that they support rather than replace orthodox medicine.*

electromagnetism – *a branch of science that deals with the relation of electricity to magnetism.*

essential oil – *a volatile and aromatic liquid (sometimes semi-solid), which generally constitutes the odorous principles of a plant. It is obtained by a process of expression or distillation from a single botanical form or species. A pure, concentrated essence taken from the plant; said to be its life force.*

flux density – *the concentration of lines of force per unit area passing from one pole to another.*

gauss – *a unit of measurement related to magnetic forces, measuring the magnetic flux density of a magnet.*

geopathic stress – *the theory that problems in the environment, particularly electromagnetism, cause malign energy fields and have a detrimental effect on health.*

magnet, ceramic – *a magnet made from synthetic material, like potter's clay, iron oxide, etc, or any other product that is first shaped and then hardened by heat and then magnetized.*

magnet, metallic – *a magnet made of metal such as iron, steel, etc, or of a mixture of metals called cast-alloy.*

magnetic field – *the space surrounding a magnet over which magnetic force is felt.*

magnetic flux – *the discharge or flow of magnetic force or the magnetic field density.*

magnetic lines of force – *continuous curve lines in the magnetic field showing the direction of the magnetic force and the value of intensity for every point surrounding a magnet.*

magnetic material –
substances or materials
such as iron, steel,
nickel, cobalt, or any
other alloy, which are
attracted by a magnet
and can retain
magnetism.

magnetization – the act
of rendering anything
magnetic or imparting
the property of
attraction and repulsion
to anything.

magnetized water – water
permeated with
magnetic force by
continuous contact with
a magnet.

meridians – channels that
run through the body,
beneath the skin, in
which the life force (chi
or qi) is carried. There are
14 main meridians
running to and from the
hands and feet to the
body and head.

pole – the extremity of any
axis about which forces
acting on it are
symmetrically disposed.
One of the two points in
a magnet, cell, or battery
having opposite
physical qualities.

North Pole – the end of
the earth's axis in the
Arctic region. The
direction in which the
north pole of a pivoted
magnet will point.

South Pole – the end of
the earth's axis in
Antarctica. The direction
in which the South pole
of a pivoted magnet will
point.

teslar – international unit
of measurement related
to magnetic forces.

yang – one aspect of the
complementary aspects
in Chinese philosophy;
reflects the active,
moving, and warmer
aspects.

yin – one aspect of the
complementary aspects
in Chinese philosophy;
reflects the passive, still,
reflective aspects.

yin/yang – Chinese
philosophy that explains
the interdependence of
all elements of nature.
These contrasting
aspects of the body and
mind must be balanced
before health and well-
being can be achieved.
Yin is the female force,
and yang is the male.

※ | # Useful suppliers

Digital Health Research Ltd
Sussex Enterprise Center
Felaw Maltings
Ipswich
IP2 8SJ
Tel: 01473 407333
Fax: 01473 407334
info@the-aegis.com
www.aegis-health.com
Aegis Electromagnetic therapy device to assist natural energy balance

Emsfield Magnetics
62 Clifton Vale Close
Clifton
Bristol
BS8 4PY
Tel: 0800 074 8753
Fax: 0117 958 5289
Magno-pulse magnetic healthcare for people and animals

Dulwich Health
130 Gipsy Hill
London
SE19 1PL
Tel: 020 8670 5883
Fax: 020 8766 6616
www.dulwichhealth.co.uk

Magnetic Therapy Ltd
Magnet House
Farm Lane
Worsley
Manchester
M28 2PG
www.magnetictherapy.co.uk

Shiatsu International
Maulak Chambers
The Centre
High Street
Halstead
Essex
CO9 2AL
www.shiatsu-international.com

Snowdon Healthcare
Pedigree House
Ambleside/Radcliffe Road
Gamston
Nottingham
NG2 6NQ
snowdenhealth@proweb.co.uk

Albert Roy Research Labs
PO Box 655
Green Cove Springs
Florida 32043
Tel: 904264 8564

BEMI
Dr. John Zimmerman
2490 W. Moana Ln.,
Reno
Nevada 89509
Tel: 702 827 9099

Nikken Inc.
10866 Wilshire Boulevard
Suite 250
Los Angeles
California 90024

✳ | Index

A

acupuncture points 7, 33, 34, 90–1, 103–21

adhesive magnets 34, 35, 48–9

air, ionized 28

alnico 13

antigens 56

anxiety 72–3

arthritis 22, 47, 64, 65

asthma 69

auras 6, 22–3, 53, 122

B

Bach remedies 72, 84–5

back pain 74

bandages 34, 60, 74

bladder meridian 114

blood

    flow 14–15, 37–9, 58, 66–7

    haemoglobin 29, 44

    oxygen 39, 44–5

    vessels 39, 40

bones 46–7, 49, 58–9

brain 19, 20, 21

bursitis 61

C

cancer 37

ceramic magnets 13, 34, 122

chi energy 7, 16

Chinese 16, 31, 90, 96–103

combined therapies 85, 87, 91

common colds 75, 86

compasses 12, 16, 93

complementary therapies 23

conception vessel 121

cramp 49, 66, 67

crystals 6, 18–19, 23

D

devices 20–1

digestive system 42–3

divining 81, 93

dreams 82–3

E

Earth 12, 28, 30, 45, 97–102

electrolytes 29

electromagnets 6, 13, 22, 24–5, 122

endorphins 20

energy 12, 18–19, 22–3, 29, 97–102, 104–21

enzymes 41, 42

experiments 27, 92–3

F

feet 35, 52, 53

ferrite 13, 34

five transformations 97–102

fluid flows 28–9, 37–9, 43, 48, 58

flux 13, 80, 123

flying dreams 82, 83

food 27, 42–3, 57, 66

fractures 58–9

G

gall bladder 118

geopathic stress 21, 30–1, 122

Gilbert, William 16

governing vessel 120

gravity 12

H

Hahnemann, Samuel 16

hands 52, 53

headaches 68–9

heart meridian 112

hemoglobin 14–15, 44

HIV 55, 56

holism 37, 85, 86–7

homeopathy 16, 34, 86–7

homes 20, 21, 27, 30

I

immune system 55, 56–7

infection 56, 57

insomnia 70

inverse square law 12, 26

iron 12, 14–15, 44, 52

J

jewelry 35

joints 46–7, 60–1

K

kidney meridian 115

L

large intestine 109

large magnets 21, 52–3

ley lines 79, 80–1, 93

liver meridian 119

lodestones 16, 17, 30, 78

lung meridian 108

lymph 37, 56–7

M

Magnetic Resonance Imaging 17

meridians 91, 104–21, 123

Merlin 78, 79, 83

Mesmer, Franz 16

metal 12, 97–102, 122

migraine 22, 25, 68, 69

Miller, Hamish 81

molecular magnets 12

morning sickness 74, 75

muscles 47

myths 78–9, 80, 83

N

neodymium iron boron 13

nervous system 41

North-seeking poles 14, 27, 48, 52, 92, 123

O

oxygen 39, 44–5

P

pacemakers 36

pain 24, 62–5, 74

Paracelsus 16

Pasteur, Louis 26

PEMFs see pulsating electromagnetic fields

pericardium 116

permanent magnets 22, 33, 34–5

pipes 28–9, 38, 39, 50

placing magnets 48

plants 26–7, 93

PMFGs see pulsed magnetic field generators

pollution 45, 69

power lines 21, 37

pregnancy 37, 75

pulmonary system 44–5

pulsating electromagnetic fields (PEMFs) 25

pulsed magnetic field generators (PMFGs) 21

R

rare-earth magnets 13

respiration 38, 44–5

rheumatism 64, 65

S

safety aspects 36–7

samarium cobalt 13

seed experiments 26

self-adhesive magnets 34, 35

self-esteem 72, 73

shiatsu 73, 88–9, 104

sleep 35, 70

small intestine 113

small magnets 48–9

South-seeking poles 14, 27, 48, 52, 92, 123

spleen meridian 110

sports injuries 60, 61

sprains 48–9

stomach 42, 110

Stonehenge 79

storage 34, 86

stress 21, 30–1, 66, 70, 85

subtle vibrational energy 22–3

suppliers 34, 124–5

surface tension 26

synovial fluid 46–7

T

tennis elbow 60–1

teslas 13, 21, 52

triple heater meridian 117

U

urinary system 39, 114

V

vibrational energy 18–19, 22–3

Vikings 16, 78

viruses 55, 56, 75

W

water 14, 26–7, 28–9, 38, 50–1, 93

wave forms 19, 22

wave generators 20–1

white blood cells 56, 57

wood element 97–102

wounds 36, 37, 51

Y

year 102, 107

yin/yang 14, 96–7, 104–21, 123

yoga 104

✳ | Acknowledgments

I particularly wish to thank my partner Joy; her total support and belief have carried me through some bad times, her wisdom and insights have strengthened the good times.

I would also like to thank Mr Julian Campbell for his patient explanations of micromagnetic devices; Magnetic Applications Ltd for all the technical information on permanent magnets; Snowden Healthcare, Magnetic Therapy Ltd, and Robinson Healthcare for providing information on the latest innovations in magnet therapy equipment.

The publisher and author would also particularly like to thank Mr Richard Whitehead from Magnetic Therapy Ltd for loaning us all the props that were used in the photoshoot for this book. A full range of Magnetic Therapy Ltd products can be viewed on www.magnetictherapy.co.uk, or write to Magnetic Therapy Ltd, Magnet House, Worsley, Manchester, England, M28 2PG.